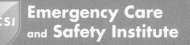

Emergency Care
and Safety Institute

First Aid

Fifth Edition

Alton Thygerson, EdD, FAWM
Medical Writer

Benjamin Gulli, MD
Medical Editor

Jon R. Krohmer, MD, FACEP
Medical Editor

American College of
Emergency Physicians®
ADVANCING EMERGENCY CARE

JONES AND BARTLETT PUBLISHERS
Sudbury, Massachusetts
BOSTON   TORONTO   LONDON   SINGAPORE

Jones and Bartlett Publishers

World Headquarters
40 Tall Pine Drive
Sudbury, MA 01776
info@jpub.com
www.ECSInstitute.org

Jones and Bartlett Publishers Canada
6339 Ormindale Way
Mississauga, Ontario L5V 1J2
Canada

Jones and Bartlett Publishers International
Barb House, Barb Mews
London W6 7PA
United Kingdom

Jones and Bartlett's books and products are available through most bookstores and online booksellers. To contact Jones and Bartlett Publishers directly, call 800-832-0034, fax 978-443-8000, or visit our website www.jbpub.com.

Substantial discounts on bulk quantities of Jones and Bartlett's publications are available to corporations, professional associations, and other qualified organizations. For details and specific discount information, contact the special sales department at Jones and Bartlett via the above contact information or send an email to specialsales@jbpub.com.

Production Credits
Chief Executive Officer: Clayton E. Jones
Chief Operating Officer: Donald W. Jones, Jr.
President, Higher Education and Professional Publishing:
  Robert W. Holland, Jr.
V.P., Sales and Marketing: William J. Kane
V.P., Production and Design: Anne Spencer
V.P., Manufacturing and Inventory Control: Therese Connell
Publisher, Public Safety Group: Kimberly Brophy
Publisher: Lawrence Newell

AAOS

AMERICAN ACADEMY OF ORTHOPAEDIC SURGEONS

Editor: Christine Emerton
Production Editor: Jenny L. McIsaac
Photo Research Manager/Photographer: Kimberly Potvin
Director of Marketing: Alisha Weisman
Interior Design: Anne Spencer
Cover Design: Kristin E. Ohlin
Composition: Auburn Associates, Inc.
Text Printing and Binding: Courier Kendallville
Cover Printing: Courier Kendallville
Cover Photograph: Rick Rykroft/AP Photo

Library of Congress Catologing-in-Publication Data

Thygerson, Alton L.
  First aid / Alton Thygerson, Benjamin Gulli ; American Academy of
Orthopaedic Surgeons, [and] American College of Emergency Physicians.— 5th ed.
    p. ; cm.
  Includes index.
  ISBN-13: 978-0-7637-4244-7 (pbk.)
  ISBN-10: 0-7637-4244-9 (pbk.)
  1. First aid in illness and injury. 2. Medical emergencies.
  [DNLM: 1. First Aid—methods. 2. Emergency. WA 292 T549fb 2006] I. Gulli, Benjamin. II. American Academy of Orthopaedic Surgeons.
III. American College of Emergency Physicians. IV. Title.
  RC86.7.T465 2006
  616.02'52—dc22
  6048
                          2006005277

Additional photographic and illustration credits appear on page 128, which constitutes a continuation of the copyright page.

Printed in the United States of America
12 11 10 09 08   10 9 8 7 6 5 4

welcome

Emergency Care and Safety Institute

Welcome to the Emergency Care and Safety Institute

Welcome to the Emergency Care and Safety Institute (ECSI), brought to you by the American Academy of Orthopaedic Surgeons (AAOS) and the American College of Emergency Physicians (ACEP).

The ECSI is an educational organization created for the purpose of delivering the highest quality training to laypersons and professionals in the areas of First Aid, CPR, AED, Bloodborne Pathogens, and related safety and health fields.

Two of the most respected names in injury, illness, and emergency medical care—AAOS and ACEP—have approved the content of our training materials.

American Academy of Orthopaedic Surgeons

About the AAOS

The AAOS provides education and practice management services for orthopaedic surgeons and allied health professionals. The AAOS also serves as an advocate for improved patient care and informs the public about the science of orthopaedics. Founded in 1933, the not-for-profit AAOS has grown from a small organization serving less than 500 members to the world's largest medical association of musculoskeletal specialists. The AAOS now serves about 24,000 members internationally.

American College of Emergency Physicians®

ADVANCING EMERGENCY CARE

About ACEP

ACEP was founded in 1968 and is the world's oldest and largest emergency medicine specialty organization. Today it represents more than 23,000 members and is the emergency medicine specialty society recognized as the acknowledged leader in emergency medicine.

ECSI Course Catalog

Individuals seeking training in ECSI subjects can choose from among various online and offline course offerings. The following courses are available through the ECSI:

First Aid, CPR, and AED Standard

CPR and AED

Professional Rescuer CPR

First Aid

Wilderness First Aid

Bloodborne Pathogens

First Responder

First Aid and CPR Online

First Aid Online

Adult CPR Online

Adult and Pediatric CPR Online

Professional Rescuer CPR Online

AED Online

Adult CPR and AED Online

Bloodborne Pathogens Online

The ECSI offers a wide range of textbooks, instructor and student support materials, and interactive technology, including online courses. Every ECSI textbook is the center of an integrated teaching and learning system that offers instructor, student, and technology resources to better support instructors and prepare students. The instructor supplements provide practical hands-on, time-saving tools like PowerPoint presentations, DVDs, and web-based distance learning resources. The student supplements are designed to help students retain the most important information and to assist them in preparing for exams. And, a key component to the teaching and learning systems are technology resources that provide interactive exercises and simulations to help students become great emergency responders.

Documents attesting to the ECSI's recognitions of satisfactory course completion will be issued to those who successfully meet the course objectives and criteria for passing the course. Written acknowledgement of a participant's successful course completion is provided in the form of a Course Completion Card, issued by the ECSI.

Visit www.ECSInstitute.org today!

resource preview

This textbook is designed to give laypersons and professionals the education and confidence they need to effectively provide emergency care. Features that will reinforce and expand on essential information include:

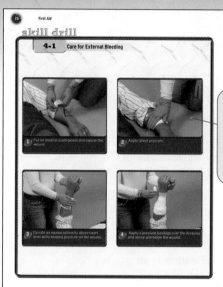

Skill Drills
Provide step-by-step explanations and visual summaries of important skills for first aiders.

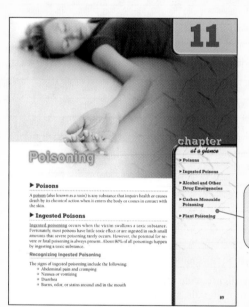

Chapter at a Glance
Guides students through the topics covered in that chapter.

Caution Boxes
Emphasize crucial actions that first aiders should or should not take while administering treatment.

FYI Boxes
Include valuable information related to the injuries or illnesses discussed in that section, including prevention tips and risk factors.

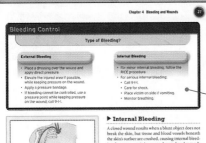

Flowcharts

Pose a central question and organize treatment options by injury or illness type.

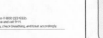

Decision Tables

Provide a concise summary of what signs first aiders should look for and what treatment steps they should take.

Prep Kit

End-of-chapter activities reinforce important concepts and improve students' comprehension.

Key Terms: List of the key terms and definitions from the chapter.

Assessment in Action: Brief case study followed by critical thinking questions that allow students to apply what they've learned.

Check Your Knowledge questions: Quiz students on the chapter's core concepts.

Background Information

▶ Why Is First Aid Important?

It's better to know first aid and not need it than to need it and not know it. Everyone should be able to perform first aid, because most people will eventually find themselves in a situation requiring it for another person or themselves.

Although a delay of just a few minutes when a person's heart stops can mean the difference between life and death, most injuries do not require lifesaving efforts. During their entire lifetimes, most people will see only one or two situations involving life-threatening conditions. Saving lives is important, but knowing what to do for less severe injuries demands greater attention and more first aid training.

▶ What Is First Aid?

First aid is the immediate care given to an injured or suddenly ill person. First aid does not take the place of proper medical care. It consists only of providing temporary assistance until competent medical care, if needed, is obtained or until the chance for recovery without medical care is assured. Most injuries and illnesses do not require medical care. **Figure 1-1** shows the leading causes

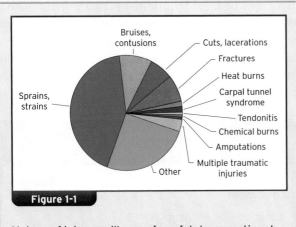

Nature of injury or illness of nonfatal occupational injuries and illnesses involving days away from work, 2003.

Figure 1-1

of nonfatal occupational injuries and illnesses in the United States. **Table 1-1** lists the leading causes of death in the United States. **Figure 1-2** compares the number of injuries resulting in deaths with the number of less severe injuries.

Properly applied, first aid may mean the difference between life and death, between a rapid recovery and a long hospitalization, or between a temporary and a permanent disability. First aid involves more than doing things for others; it also includes care that people can provide in an emergency for themselves.

▶ First Aid Supplies

The supplies in a first aid kit should be customized to include those items likely to be used on a regular basis **Figure 1-3** . A kit for the home is often different

Table 1-1 Leading Causes of Death

Rank	<1	1-4	5-9	10-14	15-24	25-34	35-44	45-54	55-64	65+	All Ages
1	Congenital Anomalies 5,621	Unintentional Injury 1,717	Unintentional Injury 1,096	Unintentional Injury 1,522	Unintentional Injury 15,272	Unintentional Injury 12,541	Unintentional Injury 16,766	Malignant Neoplasms 49,843	Malignant Neoplasms 95,692	Heart Disease 563,390	Heart Disease 685,089
2	Short Gestation 4,849	Congenital Anomalies 541	Malignant Neoplasms 516	Malignant Neoplasms 560	Homicide 5,368	Suicide 5,065	Malignant Neoplasms 15,509	Heart Disease 37,732	Heart Disease 65,060	Malignant Neoplasms 388,911	Malignant Neoplasms 556,902
3	SIDS 2,162	Malignant Neoplasms 392	Congenital Anomalies 180	Suicide 244	Suicide 3,988	Homicide 4,516	Heart Disease 13,600	Unintentional Injury 15,837	Chronic Low. Respiratory Disease 12,077	Cerebro-vascular 138,134	Cerebro-vascular 157,689
4	Maternal Pregnancy Comp. 1,710	Homicide 376	Homicide 122	Congenital Anomalies 206	Malignant Neoplasms 1,651	Malignant Neoplasms 3,741	Suicide 6,602	Liver Disease 7,466	Diabetes Mellitus 10,731	Chronic Low Respiratory Disease 109,139	Chronic Low Respiratory Disease 126,382
5	Placenta Cord Membranes 1,099	Heart Disease 186	Heart Disease 104	Homicide 202	Heart Disease 1,133	Heart Disease 3,250	HIV 5,340	Suicide 6,481	Cerebro-vascular 9,946	Alzheimer's Disease 62,814	Unintentional Injury 109,277
6	Unintentional Injury 945	Influenza & Pneumonia 163	Influenza & Pneumonia 75	Heart Disease 160	Congenital Anomalies 451	HIV 1,588	Homicide 3,110	Cerebro-vascular 6,127	Unintentional Injury 9,170	Influenza & Pneumonia 57,670	Diabetes Mellitus 74,219
7	Respiratory Distress 831	Septicemia 85	Septicemia 39	Chronic Low Respiratory Disease 81	Influenza & Pneumonia 244	Diabetes Mellitus 657	Liver Disease 3,020	Diabetes Mellitus 5,658	Liver Disease 6,428	Diabetes Mellitus 54,919	Influenza & Pneumonia 65,163
8	Bacterial Sepsis 772	Perinatal Period 79	Benign Neoplasms 38	Influenza & Pneumonia 72	Cerebro-vascular 221	Cerebro-vascular 583	Cerebro-vascular 2,460	HIV 4,442	Suicide 3,843	Nephritis 35,254	Alzheimer's Disease 63,457
9	Neonatal Hemorrhage 649	Chronic Low Respiratory Disease 55	Chronic Low Respiratory Disease 37	Benign Neoplasms 41	Chronic Low Respiratory Disease 191	Congenital Anomalies 426	Diabetes Mellitus 2,049	Chronic Low Respiratory Disease 3,537	Nephritis 3,806	Unintentional Injury 34,355	Nephritis 42,453
10	Circulatory System Disease 591	Benign Neoplasms 51	Cerebro-vascular 29	Cerebro-vascular 40	HIV 178	Influenza & Pneumonia 373	Influenza & Pneumonia 992	Viral Hepatitis 2,259	Septicemia 3,651	Septicemia 26,445	Septicemia 34,069

Source: Produced by Office of Statistics and Programming, National Center for Injury Prevention and Control, US Centers for Disease Control and Prevention. Data source: National Center for Health Statistics (NCHS) Vital Statistics Systems. Available at http://webapp.cdc.gov/sasweb/ncipc/leadcaus10.htm.

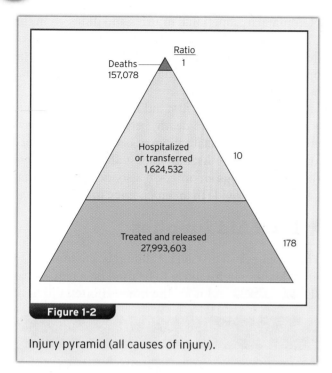

Figure 1-2

Injury pyramid (all causes of injury).

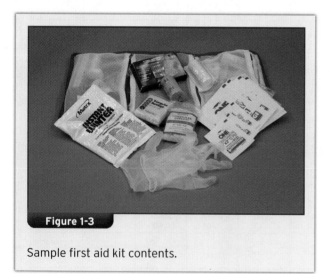

Figure 1-3

Sample first aid kit contents.

there may be local requirements that restrict the use of these items by first aiders without prior written approval. For example, teachers, activity leaders, and bus drivers in certain areas may not be able to administer these items to children without specific written permission signed by a child's parent or guardian.

Table 1-2 Sample Workplace First Aid Kit	
Equipment	**Minimum Quantity**
Adhesive strip bandages (1″ × 3″)	20
Triangular bandages (muslin, 36-40″ × 36″-40″ × 52-56″)	4
Sterile eye pads ($2\frac{1}{8}$″ × $2\frac{5}{8}$″)	2
Sterile gauze pads (4″ × 4″)	6
Sterile nonstick pads (3″ × 4″)	6
Sterile trauma pads (5″ × 9″)	2
Sterile trauma pads (8″ × 10″)	1
Sterile conforming roller gauze (2″ width)	3 rolls
Sterile conforming roller gauze (4.5″ width)	3 rolls
Waterproof tape (1″ × 5 yd)	1 roll
Porous adhesive tape (2″ × 5 yd)	1 roll
Elastic roller bandages (4″ and 6″)	1 each
Antiseptic skin wipes, individually wrapped	10
Antibiotic ointment, individual packets	6
Medical exam gloves (various sizes)	2 pairs per size
Mouth-to-barrier device (either a face mask with a one-way valve or a disposable face shield)	1
Disposable instant cold packs	2
Sealable plastic bags (quart size)	2
Padded malleable splint (SAM splint, 4″ × 36″)	1
Emergency blanket	1
Scissors	1
Tweezers	1
Biohazard waste bag (3.5 gallon capacity)	2
List of local emergency telephone numbers	1
Mini flashlight and batteries	1

from one for the workplace. A home kit may contain personal medications and a smaller number of items. A workplace kit will need more items (such as bandages) and will not include personal medications. Table 1-2 lists the basic items that should be stocked in a first aid kit for a workplace.

Although a first aid kit may have some medications, such as antihistamines and topical ointments,

▶ First Aid and the Law

Fear of lawsuits has made some people hesitant of becoming involved in emergency situations. First aiders, however, are rarely sued. Following are the legal principles that govern first aid.

Good Samaritan Laws

In most emergencies, you are not legally required to give first aid. To encourage people to assist others needing help, <u>Good Samaritan laws</u> provide protection against lawsuits. Although laws vary from state to state, Good Samaritan protection generally applies only when the rescuer is:

- Acting during an emergency
- Acting in good faith, which means he or she has good intentions
- Acting without compensation
- Not guilty of malicious misconduct or gross negligence toward the victim (intentionally deviating from established medical guidelines)

Good Samaritan laws are not a substitute for competent first aid or for staying within the scope of your training. To find out about your state's Good Samaritan laws, ask for information at your local library or ask an attorney.

Duty to Act

<u>Duty to act</u> requires an individual to provide first aid. No one is required to give first aid when no legal duty exists. Duty to act may apply in the following situations:

- *When employment requires it.* If your employer designates you as responsible for providing first aid to meet Occupational Safety and Health Administration (OSHA) requirements and you

are called to an emergency, you are required to provide first aid. Examples of occupations that involve a duty to act include law enforcement officers, park rangers, athletic trainers, lifeguards, and teachers **Figure 1-4** .

- *When a preexisting responsibility exists.* You may have a preexisting relationship with other persons that makes you responsible for them, which means you must give first aid if they need it. For example, a parent has a preexisting responsibility for a child, and a driver for a passenger.

Consent

A first aider must have the <u>consent</u> (permission) of a responsive (alert) person before providing care. The victim may give this permission verbally or with a nod of the head (<u>expressed consent</u>). Tell the victim

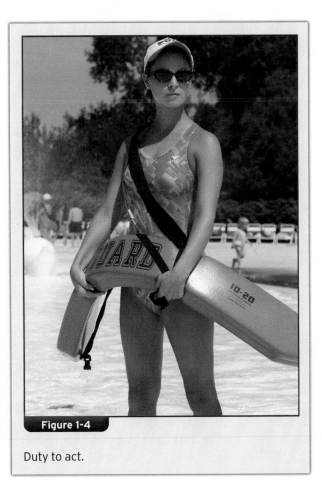

Figure 1-4

Duty to act.

your name, that you have first aid training, and what you would like to do to help.

When the victim is unresponsive (motionless), an adult who is mentally incompetent, or a child with a life-threatening condition whose parent or legal guardian is not available, first aiders should assume that <u>implied consent</u> is given. This assumes that the victim (or parent/guardian) would want care provided.

Abandonment

Once you have started first aid, do not leave the victim until another trained person takes over. Leaving the victim without help is known as <u>abandonment</u>.

Negligence

<u>Negligence</u> occurs when a victim suffers further injury or harm because the care that was given did not meet the standards expected from a person with similar training in a similar situation. Negligence involves the following:

- Having a duty to act, but either not doing so or doing so incorrectly
- Causing injury and damages

Meeting OSHA Guidelines

This chapter covers the following *OSHA Best Practices Guide: Fundamentals of a Workplace First Aid Program (2006)*:

2. Preparing to Respond to a Health Emergency
   - Understanding the legal aspects of providing first aid care, including Good Samaritan legislation, consent, abandonment, negligence, assault and battery, State Laws and regulations.

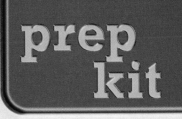

▶ Key Terms

<u>abandonment</u> Failure to continue first aid until relieved by someone with the same or higher level of training.

<u>consent</u> Permission from a victim to allow the first aider to provide care.

<u>duty to act</u> An individual's legal responsibility to provide victim care.

<u>expressed consent</u> Consent explicitly given by a victim that permits the first aider to provide care.

<u>first aid</u> Immediate care given to an injured or suddenly ill person.

<u>Good Samaritan laws</u> Laws that encourage individuals to voluntarily help an injured or suddenly ill person by minimizing the liability for errors made while rendering emergency care in good faith.

<u>implied consent</u> Consent assumed because the victim is unresponsive, mentally incompetent, or underage and has no parent or guardian present.

<u>negligence</u> Deviation from the accepted standard of care resulting in further injury to the victim.

▶ Assessment in Action

You are driving slowly looking for a house number in an unfamiliar residential area. You are attempting to deliver an important package to a customer. You see an elderly woman lying motionless at the bottom of porch stairs outside a house. You see no one else in the neighborhood, and you are alone. You quickly, but safely, stop your vehicle in front of the victim's house. As you approach the victim, you notice that her skin appears bluish.

Directions: Circle Yes if you agree with the statement, and circle No if you disagree.

Yes   No   **1.** Do you have to stop to help her?

Yes   No   **2.** You have implied consent to help this person.

Yes   No   **3.** If she does not respond to your tapping on her shoulders and shouting "Are you OK?" you can leave her and assume that someone else who is more competent or is a family member will arrive shortly to help her.

Yes   No   **4.** You decide to help. Without examining the victim you quickly straighten her legs, which suddenly causes a bone to protrude through the skin. Would this increase the likelihood of being sued?

Answers: **1.** No; **2.** Yes; **3.** No; **4.** Yes

▶ Check Your Knowledge

Directions: Circle Yes if you agree with the statement, and circle No if you disagree.

Yes   No   **1.** Because an ambulance can arrive within minutes in most locations, most people do not need to learn first aid.

Yes   No   **2.** Correct first aid can mean the difference between life and death.

Yes   No   **3.** During your lifetime, you are likely to encounter many life-threatening emergencies.

Yes   No   **4.** All injured victims need medical care.

Yes   No   **5.** Before giving first aid, you must get consent (permission) from an alert, competent adult victim.

Yes   No   **6.** If you ask an injured adult if you can help, and she says "No," you can ignore her and proceed to provide care.

Yes   No   **7.** People who are designated as first aiders by their employer must give first aid to injured employees while on the job.

Yes   No   **8.** First aiders who help injured victims are rarely sued.

Yes   No   **9.** Good Samaritan laws provide a degree of protection for first aiders who act in good faith and without compensation.

Yes   No   **10.** You are required to provide first aid to any injured or suddenly ill person you encounter.

Answers: **1.** No; **2.** Yes; **3.** No; **4.** No; **5.** Yes; **6.** No; **7.** Yes; **8.** Yes; **9.** Yes; **10.** No

2

Action at an Emergency

▶ Recognize the Emergency

The bystander is a vital link between medical care and the victim. Typically it is a bystander who first recognizes a situation as an emergency and acts to help the victim. To help in an emergency, the bystander first has to notice that something is wrong; usually, a person's appearance or behavior or the surroundings suggest that something unusual has happened.

▶ Decide to Help

At some point, everyone will have to decide whether to help another person. You will be more likely to get involved if you have previously considered the possibility of helping others. Thus, the most important time to make the decision to help is before you ever encounter an emergency.

Size Up the Scene

If you are at the scene of an emergency, take a few seconds to briefly survey the scene, considering three things:

1. *Hazards that could be dangerous to you, the victim(s), or bystanders.* Before approaching the victim(s), scan the area for immediate dangers (such

as oncoming traffic, electrical wires, or an assailant). Always ask yourself: Is the scene safe?

2. *Impression of what happened.* Is it an injury or illness, and is it severe or minor?

3. *How many people are involved.* There may be more than one victim, so look around and ask about others who might have been involved.

▶ Call 9-1-1

Laypersons sometimes make wrong decisions about calling 9-1-1. They may delay calling 9-1-1 or even bypass emergency medical services (EMS) and transport the seriously ill or injured victim to medical care in a private vehicle when an ambulance would have been better for the victim. Some employment situations require that EMS be called rather than having a layperson transport a patient. Fortunately, most injuries and sudden illnesses you encounter will not need more advanced medical care—only first aid. Nevertheless, you should know when to seek medical care.

When to Seek Medical Care

To know when to seek medical care, you must know the difference between a minor injury or illness and a life-threatening one. For example, upper abdominal pain could be indigestion, ulcers, or an early sign of a heart attack. Wheezing may be related to a person's asthma, for which the person can use his or her prescribed inhaler for quick relief, or it can be a severe, life-threatening allergic reaction to a bee sting.

Not every cut needs stitches, nor does every burn require medical care. However, it is always best to err on the side of caution. When a serious situation occurs, call 9-1-1 *first*. Do not call your doctor, the hospital, or a friend, relative, or neighbor for help before you call 9-1-1. Calling anyone else first only wastes time. Table 2-1 provides guidance on when to call 9-1-1.

How to Call 9-1-1

To receive emergency assistance in most communities, you simply dial 9-1-1. Check to see if this is true in your community. Emergency telephone numbers are usually listed on the inside front cover of telephone directories. Keep these numbers nearby or on

Table 2-1 When to Call 9-1-1

If the answer to any of the following questions is yes, or if you are unsure, call 9-1-1 or your local emergency number for help.

- Is the victim's condition life threatening?
- Could the condition get worse and become life threatening on the way to the hospital?
- Does the victim need the skills or equipment of emergency medical technicians or paramedics?
- Would distance or traffic conditions cause a delay in getting to the hospital?

The following are specific serious conditions for which 9-1-1 should also be called:

- Fainting
- Chest or abdominal pain or pressure
- Sudden dizziness, weakness, or change in vision
- Difficulty breathing or shortness of breath
- Severe or persistent vomiting
- Sudden, severe pain anywhere in the body
- Suicidal or homicidal feelings
- Bleeding that does not stop after 10 to 15 minutes of pressure
- A gaping wound with edges that do not come together
- Problems with movement or sensation following an injury
- Cuts on the hand or face
- Puncture wounds
- The possibility that foreign bodies such as glass or metal have entered a wound
- Most animal bites and all human bites
- Hallucinations and clouding of thoughts
- A stiff neck in association with a fever or a headache
- A bulging or abnormally depressed fontanel (soft spot) in infants
- Stupor or dazed behavior accompanying a high fever
- Unequal pupil size, loss of consciousness, blindness, staggering, or repeated vomiting after a head injury
- Spinal injuries
- Severe burns
- Poisoning
- Drug overdose

Source: American College of Emergency Physicians.

every telephone. Dial "0" (the operator) if you do not know the emergency number. When you call 9-1-1, the dispatcher will request certain information:

1. *The victim's location.* Give the address, names of intersecting roads, and other landmarks. Also, tell the specific location of the victim (for example, "in the basement").
2. *The phone number you are calling from and your name.* This prevents false calls and allows a dispatch center without the enhanced 9-1-1 system to call back if you are disconnected or for additional information if needed.
3. *What happened.* State the nature of the emergency (for example, "A worker fell off a ladder and is not moving").
4. *Number of persons needing help and any special conditions* (for example, "There is a liquid spilling from the truck onto the roadway").
5. *Victim's condition* (for example, "He is bleeding from the head") and any care you have provided (such as pressing on the site of the bleeding).

Do *not* hang up the phone until the dispatcher instructs you to do so. The EMS dispatcher may also tell you what to do until EMS arrives. If you send someone else to call, have the person report back to you so you can be sure the call was made.

▶ Provide Care

Often the most critical life support measures are effective only if started immediately by the nearest available person. That person usually will be a bystander.

▶ Disease Transmission

The risk of acquiring an infectious disease while providing first aid is very low. But it can be even lower if you know how to protect yourself against diseases transmitted by blood and air.

Bloodborne Diseases

Some diseases are carried by an infected person's blood (bloodborne diseases). Contact with infected blood may result in infection by one of several viruses, such as the following:

- Hepatitis B virus
- Hepatitis C virus
- Human immunodeficiency virus

Hepatitis is a viral infection of the liver. Hepatitis B virus (HBV) and hepatitis C virus (HCV) infections result in long-term liver conditions and can lead to liver cancer. Each is caused by a different virus. A vaccine is available for HBV but not for HCV. Employers are required to provide free vaccinations for employees who may be at risk for HBV (for example, health care providers).

A person infected with human immunodeficiency virus (HIV) can infect others, and those infected with HIV almost always develop acquired immunodeficiency syndrome (AIDS), which is a major cause of death worldwide. No vaccine is available to prevent HIV infection. The best defense against AIDS is to avoid becoming infected.

Airborne Diseases

Diseases transmitted through the air by coughing or sneezing (airborne diseases) include tuberculosis (TB). TB has increased in frequency and is receiving much attention. TB, which is caused by a bacteria, usually settles in the lungs and can be fatal. In most cases, a first aider will not know that a victim has TB.

Assume that any person with a cough, especially one who is in a nursing home or a shelter, may have TB. Other symptoms include fatigue, weight loss, chest pain, and coughing up blood. If a surgical mask is available, wear it or wrap a handkerchief over your nose and mouth.

Protection

In most cases, you can control the risk of exposure to diseases by wearing personal protective equipment (PPE) and by following some simple procedures. PPE blocks entry of organisms into the body. The most common type of protection involves wearing medical exam gloves **Figure 2-1**. All first aid kits should have several pairs of gloves. Because some rescuers have allergic reactions to latex, latex-free gloves (vinyl or nitrile) should be available.

Protective eyewear and a standard surgical mask may be necessary in some emergencies; first aiders ordinarily will not have or need such equipment. Mouth-to-barrier devices are recommended for cardiopulmonary resuscitation (CPR) **Figure 2-2**.

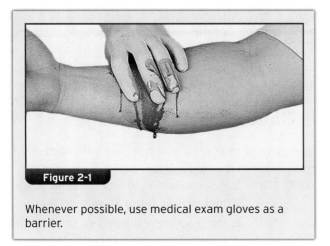

Figure 2-1

Whenever possible, use medical exam gloves as a barrier.

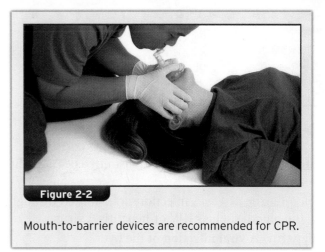

Figure 2-2

Mouth-to-barrier devices are recommended for CPR.

Always assume that *all* blood and body fluids are infected. Protect yourself even if blood or body fluids are not visible. At the workplace, PPE must be accessible, and your employer must provide training to help you choose the right PPE for your work.

First aiders can protect themselves and others against diseases by following these steps:

1. Wear appropriate PPE, such as gloves. If they are not available, put your hands in plastic bags or use waterproof material for protection.
2. If you have been trained in the correct procedures, use absorbent barriers to soak up blood or other infectious materials.
3. Clean the spill area with an appropriate disinfecting solution, such as diluted bleach (one fourth cup of bleach in a gallon of water).
4. Discard contaminated materials in an appropriate waste disposal container.
5. Wash your hands with soap and water after giving first aid.
6. If the exposure happened at work, report the incident to your supervisor. Otherwise, contact your personal physician.

▶ Rescuer Reactions

After providing care for severe injuries or illnesses, rescuers may feel an emotional letdown. Stressful events can be psychologically overwhelming and may result in a condition known as <u>post-traumatic stress disorder</u>. Its symptoms include depression and flashbacks. Discussing your feelings, fears, and reactions within 24

to 72 hours of helping at a traumatic injury scene helps prevent later emotional problems. You could discuss your feelings with a trusted friend, a mental health professional, or a member of the clergy. Quickly bringing out your feelings helps relieve personal anxieties and stress.

Meeting OSHA Guidelines

This chapter covers the following *OSHA Best Practices Guide: Fundamentals of a Workplace First Aid Program (2006)*:

2. Preparing to Respond to a Health Emergency
   • Interacting with the local EMS system;
   • Understanding the effects of stress, fear of infection, panic; how they interfere with performance; and what to do to overcome these barriers to action;
   • Learning the importance of universal precautions and body substance isolation to provide protection from bloodborne pathogens and other potentially infectious materials. Learning about personal protective equipment.
3. Assessing the Scene and the Victim(s)
   • Assessing the scene for safety, number of injured, and nature of the event;
   • Emphasizing early activation of EMS.
5. Responding to Non-Life-Threatening Emergencies
   • Wounds
      • Principles of body substance isolation, universal precautions and use of personal protective equipment.

prep kit

▶ Key Terms

airborne diseases Infections transmitted through the air, such as tuberculosis.

bloodborne diseases Infections transmitted through the blood, such as HIV or hepatitis B virus.

hepatitis A viral infection of the liver.

human immunodeficiency virus (HIV) The virus that causes acquired immunodeficiency syndrome (AIDS).

personal protective equipment (PPE) Equipment, such as medical exam gloves, used to block the entry of an organism into the body.

post-traumatic stress disorder A psychological disorder that may occur after a stressful event; symptoms include depression and flashbacks.

tuberculosis (TB) A bacterial disease that usually affects the lungs.

▶ Assessment in Action

You are rushing parts to one of your largest customer's broken machines. Because time is money, the customer is losing a lot for each hour the machine is down. It's beginning to rain. Suddenly, you see a motorcyclist skid off the highway and into a ditch. You have a cellular telephone in your car.

Directions: Circle Yes if you agree with the statement, and circle No if you disagree.

Yes   No   1. As you approach the victim, you should not be concerned about any other possible victims.

Yes   No   2. This crash scene could be dangerous.

Yes   No   3. In most communities, 9-1-1 can be used to contact the EMS.

Yes   No   4. Expect to give your name when you call 9-1-1.

Yes   No   5. If you do not know the exact address of the emergency, be prepared to give a description of the location as best as you can.

Answers: 1. No; 2. Yes; 3. Yes; 4. Yes; 5. Yes

▶ Check Your Knowledge

Directions: Circle Yes if you agree with the statement, and circle No if you disagree.

Yes   No   1. A scene survey should be done before giving first aid to an injured victim.

Yes   No   2. For a severely injured victim, call the victim's doctor before calling for an ambulance.

Yes   No   3. Dial "0" (for the telephone operator) if you do not know the emergency telephone number.

Yes   No   4. First aiders should assume that blood and all body fluids are infectious.

Yes   No   5. If you are exposed to blood while on the job, report it to your supervisor, and if off the job, to your personal physician.

Yes   No   6. First aid kits should contain medical exam gloves.

Yes   No   7. Wash your hands with soap and water after giving first aid.

Yes   No   8. Vaccinations are available for both HBV and HCV.

Yes   No   9. Medical exam gloves can be made of almost any material as long as they fit the hand well.

Yes   No   10. Tuberculosis is a bloodborne disease.

Answers: 1. Yes; 2. No; 3. Yes; 4. Yes; 5. Yes; 6. Yes; 7. Yes; 8. No; 9. No; 10. No

Finding Out What's Wrong

▶ Checking the Victim

As you approach an emergency scene, do a quick <u>scene size-up</u> to determine safety, the general type of problem (for example, whether it is an injury or illness and whether it is severe or minor), and the number of victims. If there are two or more victims, go to the quiet, motionless victim(s) first.

When you reach the victim, check to see what is wrong. Identify and correct any immediate life-threatening conditions first.

If there are no immediate threats to life, do a quick physical exam and gather information (history) about the problem.

▶ Initial Check

The <u>initial check</u> determines whether there are life-threatening problems requiring quick care. This step involves checking for the following:

- Responsiveness
- Airway
- Breathing
- Severe bleeding

It will take only seconds to complete this initial check, unless care is required at any point **Skill Drill 3-1** :

1. Determine if the victim is responsive: Call the victim in a tone of voice that is loud enough for the victim to hear. If the victim does not respond to the sound of your voice, gently tap or shake the victim's shoulder (**Step ❶**).
2. Ensure that the victim's airway is open: In the case of an unresponsive victim, open the airway by using the head tilt–chin lift maneuver (**Step ❷**).
3. Determine if the victim is breathing: Look, listen, and feel for signs of breathing (**Step ❸**).
4. Check for any obvious severe bleeding (**Step ❹**).

Check Responsiveness

If the victim is alert and talking, then breathing and heartbeat are present. Ask the victim his or her name and what happened. If the victim responds, then the victim is alert.

If the victim lies motionless, tap his or her shoulder and ask, "Are you okay?" If there is no response, the victim is considered unresponsive, and someone should call 9-1-1.

Open Airway

In an unresponsive victim, the airway must be open for breathing. If the victim is alert and able to answer questions, the airway is open. If a responsive victim cannot talk or cough forcefully, the airway is probably blocked and must be cleared. In a responsive adult or child victim, abdominal thrusts (Heimlich maneuver) can be given to clear a blocked airway.

In an unresponsive victim lying face up, open the airway using the head tilt–chin lift method. Once the victim's airway is open, the initial check can continue.

Check Breathing

In this step you check to see if the victim is breathing and, if so, if he or she is having any obvious difficulty breathing. See **Table 3-1** for breathing sounds that may indicate a problem.

With the airway of an unresponsive victim held open, look, listen, and feel for signs of breathing for 5 to 10 seconds. Look for the victim's chest to rise and

Table 3-1 Abnormal Breathing Sounds

Abnormal Sound	Possible Causes
Snoring	Airway partially blocked (usually by tongue)
Gurgling (breaths passing through liquid)	Fluids in throat
Crowing (birdlike sound)	Airway partially blocked
Wheezing	Spasm or partial obstruction in bronchi (asthma, emphysema)
Occasional, gasping breaths (known as agonal respirations)	Temporary breathing after the heart has stopped

fall. Listen for breathing sounds. Feel for escaping air on your cheek. If the victim is not breathing, you should provide two initial breaths and give CPR.

Check for Severe Bleeding

Check for severe bleeding by quickly scanning for blood up and down the body, for blood-soaked clothing, or for blood collecting on the ground or floor. If you see severe bleeding, control it with pressure. Chapter 4 covers the steps of bleeding control.

▶ Physical Exam

With the initial check complete, and no life-threatening conditions present, perform a quick <u>physical exam</u> to gather information about the victim's condition. During this time you will note the victim's signs.

- **Signs** = Conditions of the victim that you can see, feel, hear, or smell
- **Symptoms** = Things the victim feels and is able to describe, such as chest pain

For the purpose of this manual, the term *signs* is used throughout to refer to things you see, feel, hear, and smell, as well as to items the victim feels and describes.

skill drill

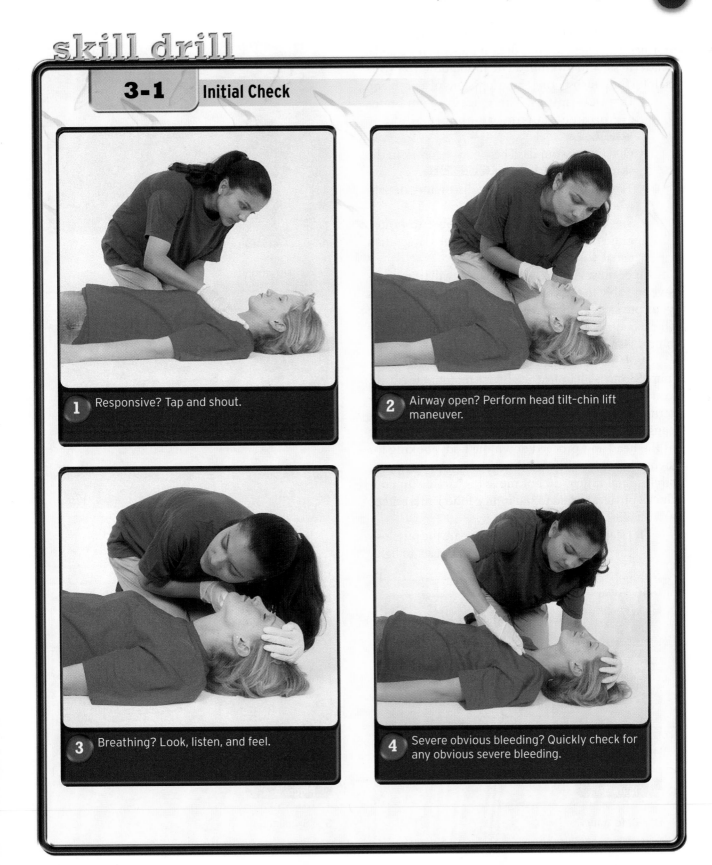

1 Responsive? Tap and shout.

2 Airway open? Perform head tilt-chin lift maneuver.

3 Breathing? Look, listen, and feel.

4 Severe obvious bleeding? Quickly check for any obvious severe bleeding.

Check the victim by looking and feeling for abnormalities. These include deformities, open wounds, tenderness, and swelling. The mnemonic <u>DOTS</u> is helpful for remembering these key signs of a problem.

- **D** = Deformities: These occur when bones are broken, causing an abnormal shape **Figure 3-1** .
- **O** = Open wounds: These cause a break in the skin and often bleeding **Figure 3-2** .
- **T** = Tenderness: Sensitivity, discomfort, or pain when touched **Figure 3-3** .
- **S** = Swelling: The body's response to injury. Fluids accumulate, so the area looks larger than usual **Figure 3-4** .

Since most victims you encounter will be responsive and able to tell you what is wrong, you can focus your physical exam on the affected area of the body (for example, an injured ankle, painful stomach, or blurry vision).

With victims who have multiple injuries (for example, from a fall from a height or a motorcycle crash), you may have to check the victim's entire body to determine the extent of the injuries. See **Table 3-2** for causes of life-threatening injuries. In this case, start at the head and proceed down the body looking for signs of problems. If you think the victim has a possible spinal injury, do not move the victim. To conduct a physical exam for an injury, follow these steps **Skill Drill 3-2** :

1. *Head:* Check for DOTS. Compare the pupils—they should be the same size and react to light.

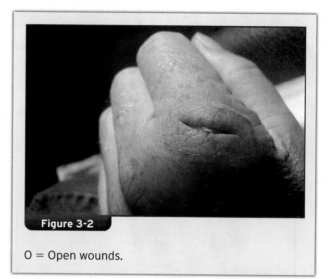

Figure 3-2

O = Open wounds.

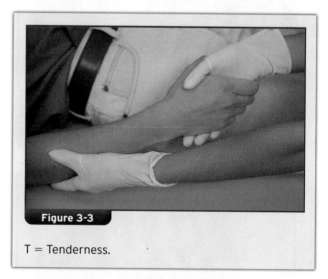

Figure 3-3

T = Tenderness.

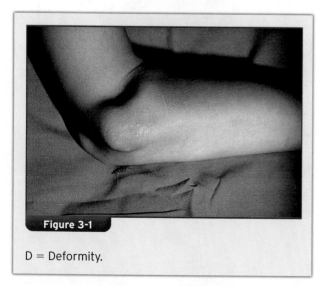

Figure 3-1

D = Deformity.

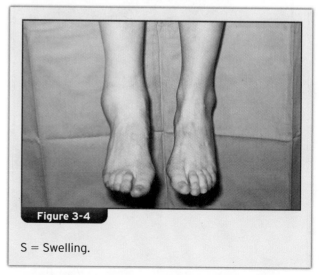

Figure 3-4

S = Swelling.

Table 3-2 Causes of Life-Threatening Injuries

Falls of more than three times the victim's height

Vehicle collisions involving ejection, a rollover, high speed, a pedestrian, a motorcycle, or a bicycle

Injuries resulting in unresponsiveness or altered mental status

Penetrations of the head, chest, or abdomen (for example, stab or gunshot wounds)

Table 3-3 Skin Color

Skin Color	Possible Cause
Pink	Normal color inside lower eyelids, inside lips, and fingernail beds of all races
Red (flushed)	Dilated blood vessels from emotional excitement, exposed to heat, high blood pressure, carbon monoxide poisoning
White (pale)	Constricted blood vessels from blood loss, shock, emotional distress
Blue (cyanotic)	Lack of oxygen in the blood and tissues from breathing or heart problems
Yellow (jaundice)	Liver disease or failure

Check the ears and nose for clear or blood-tinged fluid. Check the mouth for objects that could block the airway, such as broken teeth (Step ❶).

2. *Neck:* Check for DOTS. Look for a medical identification necklace (Step ❷).
3. *Chest:* Check for DOTS. Gently squeeze (Step ❸).
4. *Abdomen:* Check for DOTS. Gently push (Step ❹).
5. *Pelvis:* Check for DOTS. Gently push downward on the tops of the hips (Step ❺ᵃ) and inward on the sides of the hips (Step ❺ᵇ).
6. *Extremities:* Check both arms and legs for DOTS (Step ❻).
7. *Back:* If no spinal injury is suspected, turn the victim on his or her side and check for DOTS.

While checking the head, check the color, temperature, and moisture of the skin, which can provide valuable information about the victim. Table 3-3 and Table 3-4 provide more information on skin color and temperature/moisture.

Low levels of oxygen in the blood result in the skin and mucous membranes becoming blue or gray (known as <u>cyanosis</u>). This change is usually obvious in the lips

Table 3-4 Skin Temperature and Moisture

Skin Temperature/ Moisture	Possible Cause
Warm and dry	Normal
Hot and moist or dry	Excessive body heat (exposed to heat, high fever, heat stroke)
Cool and moist	Poor circulation, shock, blood loss
Cold and moist or dry	Exposed to cold and losing heat (hypothermia, frostbite)

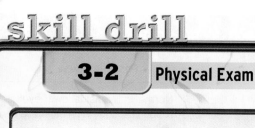
skill drill

3-2   Physical Exam

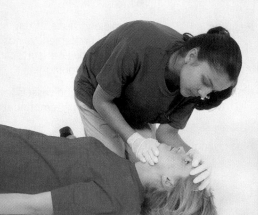

1 *Head:* Check for DOTS. Compare the pupils—they should be the same size and react to light. Check the ears and nose for clear or blood-tinged fluid. Check the mouth for objects that could block the airway, such as broken teeth.

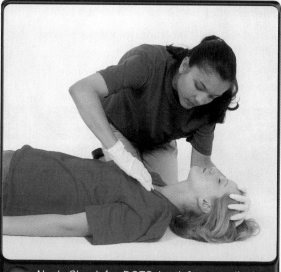

2 *Neck:* Check for DOTS. Look for a medical identification necklace.

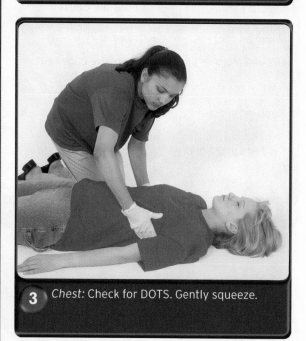

3 *Chest:* Check for DOTS. Gently squeeze.

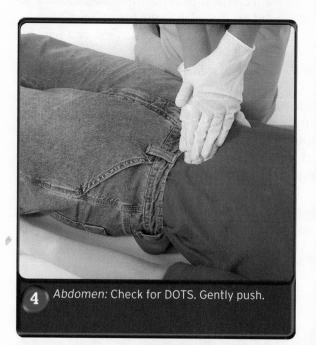

4 *Abdomen:* Check for DOTS. Gently push.

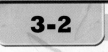

skill drill

3-2 Physical Exam Continued

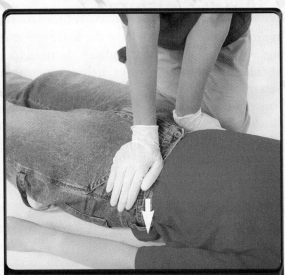

5a *Pelvis:* Check for DOTS. Gently push downward on the tops of the hips.

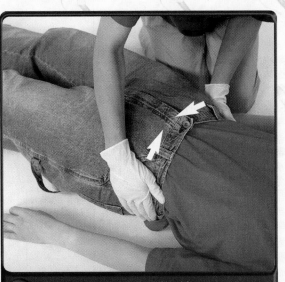

5b Gently press inward on the hips.

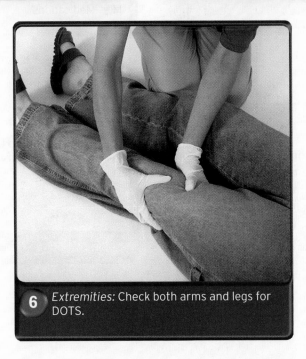

6 *Extremities:* Check both arms and legs for DOTS.

CAUTION

When doing a physical exam:
DO NOT aggravate injuries.
DO NOT move a victim with a possible spinal injury.

FYI

Medical Identification Tags

Remember to look for a medical identification tag, which may be beneficial for identifying allergies, medications, or medical history Figure 3-5 .

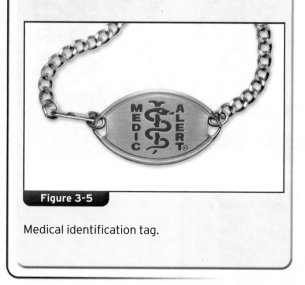

Figure 3-5

Medical identification tag.

and skin of light-skinned persons. In darkly pigmented persons, it can be seen in the mouth's mucous membranes, nail beds, and inner lining of the eyelids.

A medical identification tag, worn as a necklace or as a bracelet, contains the wearer's medical problem(s) and a 24-hour telephone number that offers, in case of an emergency, access to the victim's medical history plus names of doctors and close relatives. Necklaces and bracelets are durable, instantly recognizable, and less likely than cards to be separated from the victim in an emergency.

▶ SAMPLE History

An alert victim may provide information that indicates what is wrong and can indicate the need for first aid. The mnemonic SAMPLE helps you remember what information to gather Table 3-5 . If the victim is unresponsive, you may be able to obtain a history from family, friends, or bystanders. As with the physical exam, gathering this information is secondary if you are dealing with a life-threatening condition.

Table 3-5   SAMPLE History

Description	Questions
S = Signs	"What's wrong?"
A = Allergies	"Are you allergic to anything?"
M = Medications	"Are you taking any medications? What are they for?"
P = Past medical history	"Have you had this problem before? Do you have other medical problems?"
L = Last oral intake	"When did you last eat or drink anything?"
E = Events leading up to the illness or injury	Injury: "How did you get hurt?"
	Illness: "What were you doing before the illness started?"

▶ What to Do Until EMS Arrives

The initial check, physical exam, and SAMPLE history are done quickly so that injuries and illnesses can be identified and appropriate first aid provided.

If possible, record information found during this process and provide this information to arriving EMS personnel. Recheck the victim's condition every few minutes until EMS personnel arrive. Record any changes in the victim's condition.

Meeting ○SHA Guidelines

This chapter covers the following *OSHA Best Practices Guide: Fundamentals of a Workplace First Aid Program (2006):*

3. Assessing the Scene and the Victim(s)
   - Assessing the scene for safety, number of victims, and nature of the event;
   - Assessing each victim for responsiveness, airway patency (blockage), breathing, circulation, and medical alert tags;
   - Taking a victim's history at the scene, including determining the mechanism of injury;
   - Performing a logical head-to-toe check for injuries;
   - Stressing the need to continuously monitor the victim;
   - Emphasizing early activation of EMS.

prep kit

▶ Key Terms

<u>cyanosis</u> Low levels of oxygen in the blood that result in the skin and mucous membranes becoming blue or gray.

<u>DOTS</u> The mnemonic for remembering key signs of a problem: deformities, open wounds, tenderness, and swelling.

<u>initial check</u> The first step in dealing with an emergency situation; this step determines whether there are life-threatening problems requiring quick care.

<u>medical identification tag</u> A bracelet or necklace that notes the wearer's medical problem(s) and a 24-hour telephone number for emergency access to the victim's medical history plus names of doctors and close relatives.

<u>physical exam</u> Process of gathering information about the victim's condition by noting the victim's signs.

<u>SAMPLE</u> The mnemonic for remembering key information about a patient's history: symptoms, allergies, medications, past medical history, last oral intake, and events leading up to the injury or illness.

<u>scene size-up</u> Quick survey of an emergency scene to determine whether there are life-threatening problems requiring quick care.

▶ Assessment in Action

A coworker calls to report that someone has fallen from a ladder while changing overhead lighting. As a company-designated first aider, you respond and see people gathered around the victim. You find the employee lying on the floor motionless. You notice that he wears a medical identification bracelet.

Directions: Circle Yes if you agree with the statement, and circle No if you disagree.

Yes   No   1. After confirming that the scene is safe, you next check the medical identification bracelet as a clue for finding out what's wrong.

Yes   No   2. If he was unresponsive, you would first look at and feel his legs for a broken bone.

Yes   No   3. If he was responsive, you would next gather his health history.

Yes   No   4. The physical exam should be started at the victim's head.

Yes   No   5. A medical identification tag lists the victim's medical problem.

Answers: 1. No; 2. No; 3. No; 4. Yes; 5. Yes

▶ Check Your Knowledge

Directions: Circle Yes if you agree with the statement, and circle No if you disagree.

Yes   No   1. The purpose of an initial check is to find life-threatening conditions.

Yes   No   2. A quiet, motionless victim may indicate a breathing problem.

Yes   No   3. Most injured victims require a complete physical exam.

Yes   No   4. For a physical exam, you usually begin at the head and work down the body.

Yes   No   5. If the victim is not breathing, give two breaths before giving chest compression.

Yes   No   6. The mnemonic DOTS helps in remembering what information to obtain about the victim's history that may be useful.

Yes   No   7. For all injured and suddenly ill persons, look for a medical identification tag during a physical exam.

Yes   No   8. The mnemonic SAMPLE can remind you how to examine an area for signs of an injury.

Yes   No   9. If there is more than one victim, go to the quiet, motionless victim first.

Yes   No   10. A gurgling sound heard while checking for breathing indicates possible fluid in the throat.

Answers: 1. Yes; 2. Yes; 3. No; 4. Yes; 5. Yes; 6. No; 7. Yes; 8. No; 9. Yes; 10. Yes

Bleeding and Wounds

▶ External Bleeding

External bleeding refers to when blood can be seen coming from an open wound. The term <u>hemorrhage</u> refers to a large amount of bleeding in a short time.

Recognizing External Bleeding

Injuries damage blood vessels and cause bleeding. The three types of bleeding relate to the type of blood vessel that is damaged: capillary, vein, or artery **Figure 4-1** .

- <u>Capillary bleeding</u> oozes from a wound steadily but slowly. It is the most common type of bleeding and easiest to control.
- <u>Venous bleeding</u> flows steadily. Because it is under less pressure, it does not spurt and is easier to control.
- <u>Arterial bleeding</u> spurts with each heartbeat. The pressure that causes the blood to spurt also makes this type of bleeding difficult to control. This is the most serious type of bleeding because a large amount of blood can be lost in a very short time.

There are several types of open wounds **Figure 4-2A–F** :

- *Abrasion:* The top layer of skin is removed, with little blood loss. Other names for an abrasion are *scrape, road rash,* and *rug burn.*

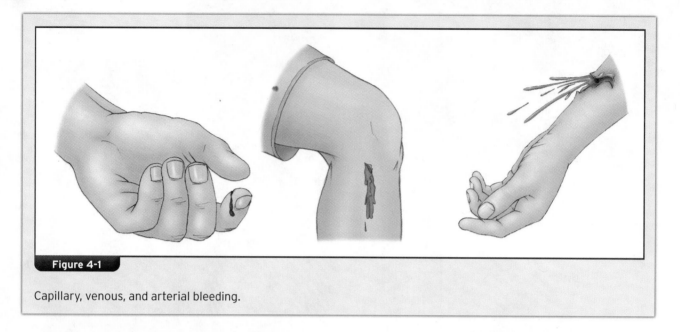

Figure 4-1

Capillary, venous, and arterial bleeding.

- *Laceration:* Cut skin with jagged edges. This type of wound is usually caused by a forceful tearing away of skin tissue.
- *Incision:* A cut with smooth edges, such as a knife or paper cut.
- *Puncture:* Injury from a sharp, pointed object (such as a knife, ice pick, or bullet). The penetrating object can damage internal organs. The risk of infection is high. The object causing the injury may remain embedded (impaled) in the wound.
- *Avulsion:* A piece of skin torn loose and hanging from the body.

- *Amputation:* The cutting or tearing off of a body part.

Care for External Bleeding

Care for external bleeding involves controlling the bleeding and protecting the wound from further injury **Skill Drill 4-1** :

1. Protect yourself against disease by wearing medical exam gloves. If they are not available, use several layers of gauze pads, clean cloths, plastic wrap, a plastic bag, or waterproof material.

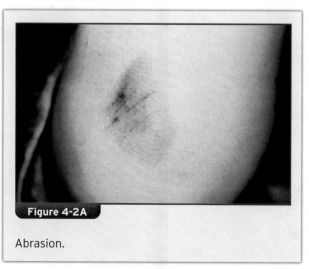

Figure 4-2A

Abrasion.

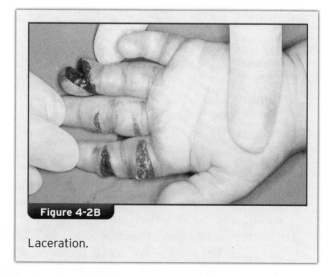

Figure 4-2B

Laceration.

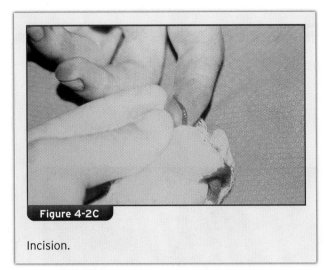

Figure 4-2C

Incision.

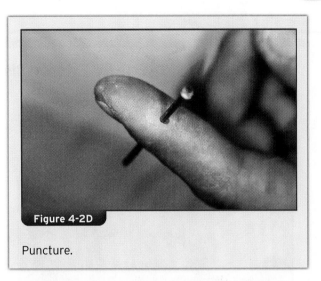

Figure 4-2D

Puncture.

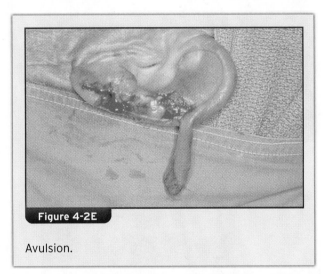

Figure 4-2E

Avulsion.

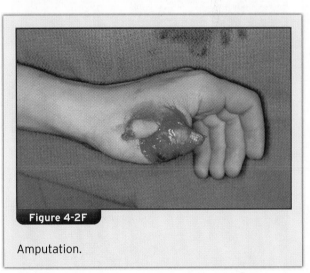

Figure 4-2F

Amputation.

2. Expose the wound by removing or cutting the clothing to find the source of the bleeding (**Step ❶**).

3. Place a dressing, such as a sterile gauze pad or a clean cloth, over the wound and apply direct pressure with your hand (**Step ❷**). This stops most bleeding.

4. If the victim is bleeding from an arm or leg, elevate the injured area above heart level to reduce blood flow as you continue to apply pressure (**Step ❸**).

5. To free you to attend to other injuries, apply a pressure bandage to hold the dressing on the wound. Wrap a roller gauze bandage in a spiral pattern tightly over the dressing and above

and below the wound (**Step ❹**).

6. If blood soaks through the dressing and bandage, do not remove the old ones. Apply an additional dressing and pressure bandage on top of the first one.

7. If the bleeding still cannot be controlled, apply pressure at a pressure point while keeping pressure on the wound. A pressure point is where an artery near the skin's surface passes close to a bone, against which it can be compressed. The most accessible pressure points on both sides of the body are the brachial pressure point on the inside of the upper arm and the femoral pressure point in the groin **Figure 4-3**.

skill drill

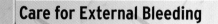

4-1   **Care for External Bleeding**

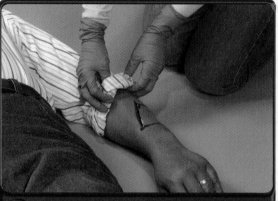

1 Put on medical exam gloves and expose the wound.

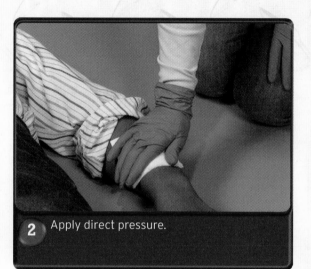

2 Apply direct pressure.

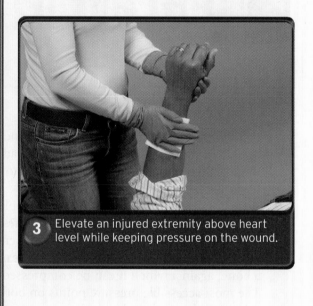

3 Elevate an injured extremity above heart level while keeping pressure on the wound.

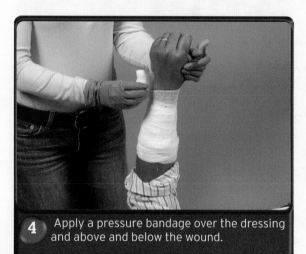

4 Apply a pressure bandage over the dressing and above and below the wound.

Bleeding Control

Type of Bleeding?

External Bleeding

- Place a dressing over the wound and apply direct pressure.
- Elevate the injured area if possible, while keeping pressure on the wound.
- Apply a pressure bandage.
- If bleeding cannot be controlled, use a pressure point while keeping pressure on the wound; call 9-1-1.

Internal Bleeding

- For minor internal bleeding, follow the RICE procedure.
- For serious internal bleeding:
  - Call 9-1-1.
  - Care for shock.
  - Place victim on side if vomiting.
  - Monitor breathing.

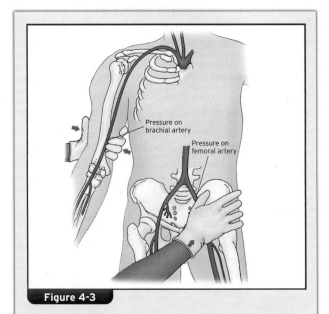

Pressure on brachial artery

Pressure on femoral artery

Figure 4-3

Proper hand positions for applying pressure on brachial and femoral arteries.

CAUTION

Once the wound has been cared for, wash your hands with soap and water, even if you used medical exam gloves.

DO NOT use direct pressure on an eye injury, a wound with an embedded object, or a skull fracture.

▶ Internal Bleeding

A closed wound results when a blunt object does not break the skin, but tissue and blood vessels beneath the skin's surface are crushed, causing internal bleeding. In some cases it is easy to detect closed wounds from the bruising that often occurs. In other cases, a closed wound can be difficult to detect but can still be life threatening.

Recognizing Internal Bleeding

The signs of internal bleeding may appear quickly or take days to appear:

- Bruising
- Painful, tender area
- Vomiting or coughing up blood
- Stool that is black or contains bright red blood

Care for Internal Bleeding

For minor internal bleeding (such as a bruise on the leg from bumping into the corner of a table), follow the steps of the RICE procedure:

1. Rest the injured area.
2. Apply an ice or cold pack over the injury.
3. Compress the injured area by applying an elastic bandage.
4. Elevate an injured arm or leg, if it is not broken.

The RICE procedure is presented in more detail in Chapter 9.

To care for serious internal bleeding, follow these steps:

1. Call 9-1-1.
2. Care for shock by raising the victim's legs 6 to 12 inches, and cover the victim to maintain warmth. See Chapter 5 for more information on shock.
3. If vomiting occurs, roll the victim onto his or her side to keep the airway clear.
4. Monitor breathing.

> **CAUTION**
>
> DO NOT give a victim anything to eat or drink. It could cause nausea and vomiting, which could result in aspiration. Food or liquids could cause complications if surgery is needed.

▶ Wound Care

A minor wound should be cleaned to help prevent infection. Wound cleaning usually restarts bleeding by disturbing the clot, but it should be done anyway. For severe bleeding, leave the pressure bandage in place until the victim can get medical care. To clean a shallow wound:

1. Wash the wound with soap and water.
2. Flush the wound with running water under pressure.
3. Remove small objects that are not flushed out with sterile tweezers.
4. If bleeding restarts, apply direct pressure over the wound.
5. Apply an antibiotic ointment.
6. Cover the area with a sterile and, if possible, nonstick dressing. Change the dressing and bandage periodically.
7. Seek medical care for a wound with a high risk for infection (such as an animal bite or a puncture).

> **CAUTION**
>
> DO NOT pull a scab loose to change the dressing. If a sticking dressing must be removed, soak it in warm water to help soften the scab and make removal easier.

▶ Wound Infection

Any wound, large or small, can become infected **Figure 4-4** . Seek medical care for infected wounds.

The signs that a wound may be infected include the following:

- Swelling and redness around the wound
- A sensation of warmth
- Throbbing pain
- Pus discharge
- Fever
- Swelling of lymph nodes
- Red streaks leading from the wound toward the heart

Tetanus

Tetanus is caused by a bacterium that can produce a powerful poisonous toxin when it enters a wound. The toxin causes contractions of certain muscle groups, particularly in the jaw. There is no known cure for the toxin.

Because of this danger, everyone needs an initial series of vaccinations to defend against the toxin. A booster shot every 10 years is sufficient to maintain immunity, although anyone with a dirty wound or an animal bite should get a booster shot right away. Tetanus immunization shots must be given within 72 hours of the injury to be effective.

▶ Special Wounds

This section addresses two special wounds: amputations and embedded (impaled) objects.

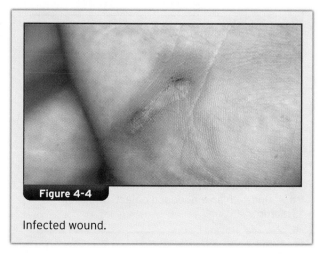

Figure 4-4

Infected wound.

Amputations

The loss of a body part is a devastating injury that requires immediate medical care. To care for an amputation **Figure 4-5** :

1. Call 9-1-1.
2. Control bleeding.
3. Care for shock.
4. Recover the amputated part and wrap it in dry sterile gauze or a clean cloth.
5. Place the wrapped amputated part in a plastic bag or other waterproof container.
6. Keep the part cool (for example, on an ice or cold pack), but do not freeze.

FYI

Cooling Amputated Parts

Amputated body parts that remain uncooled for more than 6 hours have little chance of survival; 18 hours is probably the maximum time allowable for a part that has been cooled properly. Muscles without blood lose viability within 4 to 6 hours.

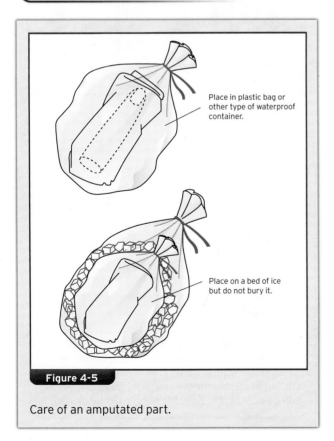

Place in plastic bag or other type of waterproof container.

Place on a bed of ice but do not bury it.

Figure 4-5

Care of an amputated part.

Embedded (Impaled) Objects

Objects such as glass, knives, and nails can be embedded (impaled) in the body **Figure 4-6** . To care for these wounds:

1. Expose the area. Remove or cut away clothing surrounding the injury.
2. Do not remove or move the object. Movement of any kind could produce additional bleeding and tissue damage.
3. Control any bleeding with pressure around the object.
4. Stabilize the object with bulky dressings or clean cloths around the object.
5. Shorten the object only if necessary.

▶ Wounds That Require Medical Care

It can be difficult to determine which wounds require a trip to the emergency department. These guidelines identify which wounds need emergency medical care.

- Wounds that will not stop bleeding after 5 minutes of applying direct pressure.
- Long or deep cuts that need stitches.
- Cuts over a joint.
- Cuts that may impair function of a body area such as an eyelid or lip.
- Cuts that remove all of the layers of the skin, such as those from slicing off the tip of a finger.
- Cuts from an animal or human bite.

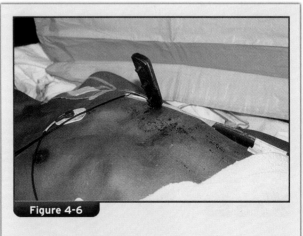

Figure 4-6

Embedded (impaled) object in the chest.

- Cuts that have damaged underlying nerves, tendons, or joints.
- Cuts over a possible broken bone.
- Cuts caused by a crushing injury.
- Cuts with an object embedded in them.
- Cuts caused by a metal object or a puncture wound.

Call 9-1-1 immediately if:

- Bleeding from the cut does not slow during the first 15 minutes of steady direct pressure.
- Signs of shock occur.
- Breathing is difficult because of a cut to the neck or chest.
- A deep cut to the abdomen causes moderate to severe pain.
- A cut to the eyeball.
- A cut amputates or partially amputates an extremity.

▶ Dressings and Bandages

First aid kits include dressings and bandages to be used when controlling bleeding and caring for wounds. A **dressing** is a covering that is placed directly over a wound to help absorb blood, prevent infection, and protect the wound from further injury. Dressings come in different shapes, sizes, and types. Dressings can be gauze pads (for example, 2- or 4-inch square or larger) used to cover larger wounds, or adhesive strips such as Band-Aids, which are dressings combined with a bandage for small cuts or scrapes **Figure 4-7** .

A **bandage**, such as a roll of gauze, is often used to cover a dressing to keep it in place on the wound and to apply pressure to help control the bleeding. Like dressings, bandages also come in different shapes, sizes, and material **Figure 4-8** . Elastic bandages can be used to provide support and stability for an extremity or joint and to reduce swelling.

When commercial bandages are unavailable, you can improvise bandages from neckties, bandanas, or strips of cloth torn from a sheet or other similar material.

When applying a bandage, do not apply it so tightly that it restricts blood circulation. The signs that a bandage is too tight are as follows:

- Blue tinge to the fingernails or toenails
- Blue or pale skin
- Tingling or loss of sensation
- Coldness of the extremity

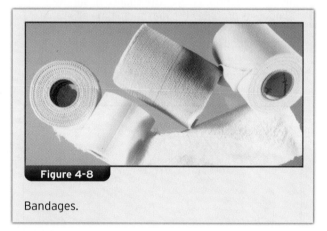

Figure 4-8

Bandages.

FYI

Sutures (Stitches)

If sutures are needed, they should be placed by a physician, usually within 6 to 8 hours of the injury. Suturing wounds allows faster healing, reduces infection, and lessens scarring.

Some wounds do not usually require sutures:

- Wounds in which the skin's cut edges tend to fall together
- Shallow cuts less than 1 inch long

Rather than close a gaping wound with butterfly bandages, cover the wound with sterile gauze. Closing the wound might trap bacteria inside, resulting in an infection. In most cases, a physician can be reached in time for sutures to be placed.

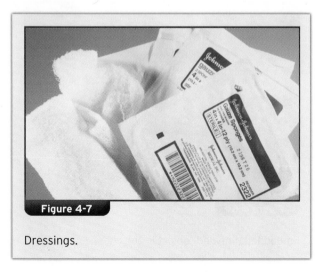

Figure 4-7

Dressings.

▶ Bleeding

What to Look For

External bleeding
- Blood coming from an open wound

Internal bleeding
- Bruising
- Painful, tender area
- Vomiting or coughing up blood
- Stool that is black or contains bright red blood

What to Do

1. Protect against blood contact.
2. Place sterile dressing over wound and apply pressure.
3. Elevate the injured area if possible.
4. Apply a pressure bandage.
5. If bleeding cannot be controlled, apply pressure to a pressure point.

Minor internal bleeding:
1. Use RICE procedures:
   - R = Rest
   - I = Ice or cold pack
   - C = Compress the area with elastic bandage
   - E = Elevate the injured extremity

Serious internal bleeding:
1. Call 9-1-1.
2. Care for shock.
3. If vomiting occurs, roll the victim onto side.

▶ Wounds

What to Look For

Wound care

What to Do

1. Wash with soap and water.
2. Flush with running water under pressure.
3. Remove remaining small object(s).
4. If the bleeding restarts, apply pressure on wound.
5. Apply antibiotic ointment.
6. Cover with sterile or clean dressing.
7. For wounds with a high risk for infection, seek medical care for cleaning, possible tetanus booster, and closing.

Wound infection
- Swelling and redness around the wound
- Sensation of warmth
- Throbbing pain
- Pus discharge
- Fever
- Swelling of lymph nodes
- Red streaks leading from the wound toward the heart

1. Seek medical care.

Amputation
- Loss of a body part

1. Call 9-1-1.
2. Control bleeding.
3. Care for shock.
4. Recover amputated part(s) and wrap in sterile or clean dressing.
5. Place wrapped part(s) in a plastic bag or waterproof container.
6. Keep part(s) cool.

Embedded (impaled) object
- Object remains in wound

1. Do not remove object.
2. Control bleeding with pressure around the object.
3. Stabilize the object with bulky dressings or clean cloths.

prep kit

▶ Key Terms

arterial bleeding Bleeding from an artery; this type of bleeding tends to spurt with each heartbeat.

bandage Used to cover a dressing to keep it in place on the wound and to apply pressure to help control bleeding.

capillary bleeding Bleeding that oozes from a wound steadily but slowly.

dressing A sterile gauze pad or clean cloth covering placed over an open wound.

hemorrhage A large amount of bleeding in a short time.

venous bleeding Bleeding from a vein; this type of bleeding tends to flow steadily.

▶ Assessment in Action

A 25-year-old construction worker has been badly cut on his thigh by a circular power saw. The cut is approximately 5 inches long, and blood is spurting from the wound.

Directions: Circle Yes if you agree with the statement, and circle No if you disagree.

Yes No **1.** This victim is experiencing venous bleeding.

Yes No **2.** You should be certain to wash this wound with soap and water.

Yes No **3.** Direct pressure should stop the bleeding.

Yes No **4.** Treat the victim for shock.

Yes No **5.** The type of bleeding experienced by this man is the most common type.

Answers: 1. No; 2. No; 3. Yes; 4. Yes; 5. No

▶ Check Your Knowledge

Directions: Circle Yes if you agree with the statement, and circle No if you disagree.

Yes No **1.** Most cases of bleeding require more than direct pressure to stop the bleeding.

Yes No **2.** Remove any blood-soaked dressings before applying additional ones.

Yes No **3.** Whenever elevating an arm or leg to control bleeding, you should also keep applying pressure on the wound.

Yes No **4.** If a bleeding arm wound is not controlled through direct pressure, elevation, and pressure bandaging, apply pressure to the brachial artery.

Yes No **5.** Dressings are placed directly on a wound.

Yes No **6.** Care for an amputated part by placing it in a container of water to keep it moist and clean.

Yes No **7.** Dressings should be sterile or as clean as possible.

Yes No **8.** Antibiotic ointments can be placed on any open wound.

Yes No **9.** Keep an amputated part packed in ice to preserve it.

Yes No **10.** It is important to remove impaled objects because they could be driven in deeper.

Answers: 1. No; 2. No; 3. Yes; 4. Yes; 5. Yes; 6. No; 7. Yes; 8. No; 9. No; 10. No

Meeting OSHA Guidelines

This chapter covers the following *OSHA Best Practices Guide: Fundamentals of a Workplace First Aid Program (2006)*:

4. Responding to Life-Threatening Emergencies
   • Controlling bleeding with direct pressure.
   • Responding to Medical Emergencies
     • Impaled object.
5. Responding to Non-Life-Threatening Emergencies
   • Wounds
     • Assessment and first aid for wounds including abrasions, cuts, lacerations, punctures, avulsions, amputations and crush injuries;
     • Principles of wound care, including infection precautions;
     • Principles of body substance isolation, universal precautions and use of personal protective equipment.
   • Musculoskeletal Injuries
     • Appropriate handling of amputated body parts.

Shock

▶ Shock

<u>Shock</u> occurs when the body's tissues do not receive enough oxygenated blood. Do not confuse this with an electric shock or "being shocked," as in being scared or surprised. To understand shock, think of the circulatory system as having three components: a working pump (the heart), a network of pipes (the blood vessels), and an adequate amount of fluid (the blood) pumped through the pipes. Damage to any of the components can deprive tissues of oxygen-rich blood and produce the condition known as shock.

Recognizing Shock

The signs of shock include the following:
- Altered mental status:
  - Agitation
  - Anxiety
  - Restlessness
  - Confusion
- Pale, cold, and clammy skin, lips, and nail beds
- Nausea and vomiting

- Rapid breathing
- Unresponsiveness (when shock is severe)

Care for Shock

Even if there are no signs of shock, you should still treat seriously injured and suddenly ill victims for shock.

1. Place the victim on his or her back.
2. Raise the legs 6 to 12 inches (if spinal injury is not suspected). Raising the legs allows the blood to drain from the legs back to the heart **Figure 5-1**.
3. Place blankets under and over the victim to keep the victim warm.

Other positions may be used in shock when other conditions are present **Figure 5-2A–D**.

▶ Anaphylaxis

A life-threatening breathing emergency can result from a severe allergic reaction called <u>anaphylaxis</u>. This reaction happens when a substance to which the victim is very sensitive enters the body. It can be deadly within minutes if untreated. Many of the deaths are caused by the inability to breathe because swollen airway passages block air to the lungs. The most common causes of anaphylaxis include the following:

- Medications (for example, penicillin and related drugs, aspirin, sulfa drugs)
- Food (for example, nuts, especially peanuts; eggs; shellfish)

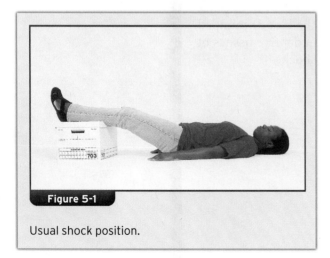

Figure 5-1

Usual shock position.

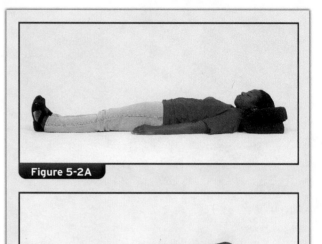

Figure 5-2A

Figure 5-2B

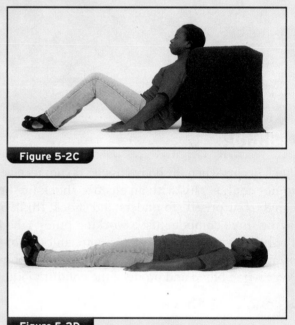

Figure 5-2C

Figure 5-2D

Other positions that may be used in certain cases of shock. **A.** For a victim with head injury, elevate the head (if spinal injury is not suspected). **B.** Position an unresponsive or stroke victim in the recovery position. **C.** Use a half-sitting position for victims with breathing difficulties, chest injuries, or a heart attack. **D.** Keep the victim flat if a spinal injury or leg fracture is suspected.

- Insect stings (for example, honeybee, yellow jacket, wasp, hornet, fire ant)
- Plants (for example, inhaled pollen)

Recognizing Anaphylaxis

The most common signs of anaphylaxis include the following:
- Breathing difficulty—shortness of breath and wheezing
- Skin reaction—itching or burning skin, especially over the face and upper part of the chest, with rash or hives
- Swelling of the tongue, mouth, or throat

Other signs of anaphylaxis are as follows:
- Sneezing, coughing
- Tightness in the chest
- Blueness around lips and mouth
- Dizziness
- Nausea and vomiting

Care for Anaphylaxis

To care for anaphylaxis:
1. Call 9-1-1.
2. Determine if the victim has medication for allergic reactions. If the victim has a prescribed epinephrine auto-injector **Figure 5-3**, help the victim use it. If you are assisting with or using an auto-injector, follow these steps **Skill Drill 5-1**:
   a. Remove the safety cap. The auto-injector is now ready for use **(Step ❶)**.
   b. Support the victim's thigh and place the black tip of the auto-injector lightly against the outer thigh.
   c. Using a quick motion, push the auto-injector firmly against the thigh and hold it in place for several seconds **(Step ❷)**. This will inject the medication.

d. Remove the auto-injector from the thigh. Carefully reinsert the used auto-injector, needle first, into the carrying tube **(Step ❸)**. A small amount of medication will remain in the device, but the device cannot be reused.
3. Keep a responsive victim sitting up to help breathing. Place an unresponsive victim on his or her side.

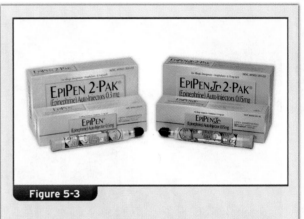

Figure 5-3

Prescribed epinephrine auto-injectors.

Meeting OSHA Guidelines

This chapter covers the following *OSHA Best Practices Guide: Fundamentals of a Workplace First Aid Program (2006)*:

4. Responding to Life-Threatening Emergencies
   - Recognizing the signs and symptoms of shock and providing first aid for shock due to illness or injury
5. Responding to Non-Life-Threatening Emergencies
   - Bites and Stings
     - Instruction in first aid treatment of anaphylactic shock

skill drill

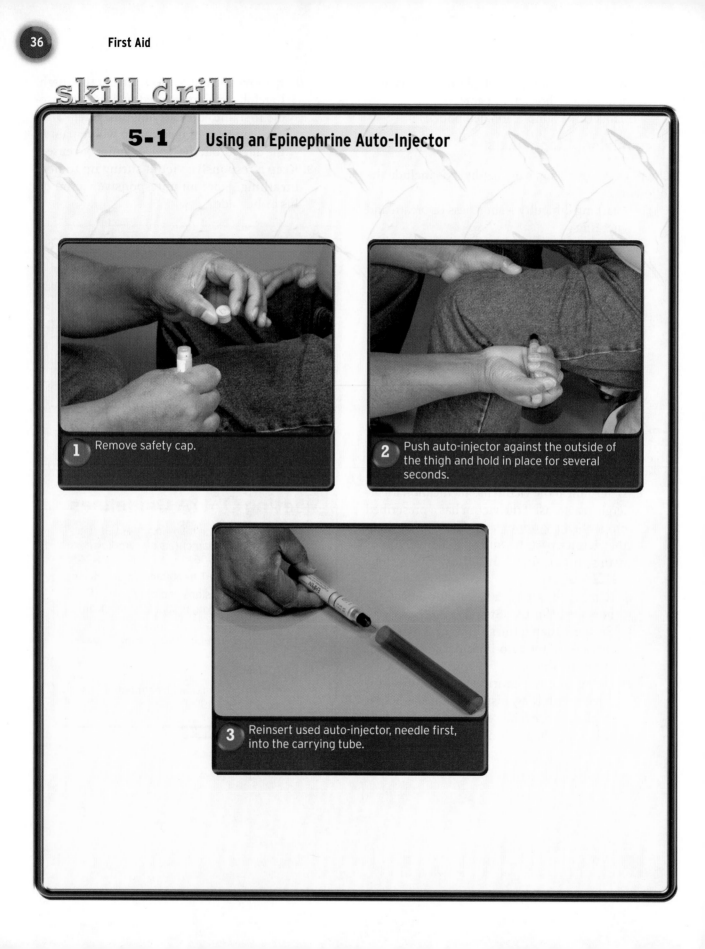

5-1 Using an Epinephrine Auto-Injector

1 Remove safety cap.

2 Push auto-injector against the outside of the thigh and hold in place for several seconds.

3 Reinsert used auto-injector, needle first, into the carrying tube.

▶ Shock and Anaphylaxis

What to Look For

What to Do

Shock
- Altered mental status (anxiety, restlessness)
- Pale, cold, and clammy skin, lips, and nail beds
- Nausea and vomiting
- Rapid breathing

1. Place the victim on his or her back and raise the legs 6 to 12 inches. Other positions are used for other conditions.
2. Place blankets under and over the victim to keep the victim warm.

Anaphylaxis
- Breathing difficulty
- Skin reaction
- Swelling of the tongue, mouth, or throat
- Sneezing, coughing
- Tightness in the chest
- Blueness around lips and mouth
- Dizziness
- Nausea and vomiting

1. Call 9-1-1.
2. Determine if victim has a prescribed epinephrine auto-injector and help the victim use it.
3. Keep a responsive victim sitting up to help breathing. Place an unresponsive victim on his or her side.

prep kit

▶ Key Terms

anaphylaxis A life-threatening allergic reaction.

epinephrine auto-injector Prescribed device used to administer an emergency dose of epinephrine to a victim experiencing anaphylaxis.

shock Inadequate tissue oxygenation resulting from serious injury or illness.

▶ Assessment in Action

A woman was working in her garden on a warm summer day. She unintentionally disturbed a nest of yellow jackets and was stung several times on her face and neck. She has begun coughing and wheezing. She complains that she is dizzy and having difficulty breathing. You notice that her face is swelling.

Directions: Circle Yes if you agree with the statement, and circle No if you disagree.

Yes   No   **1.** Breathing difficulty and swelling may be signs of a severe allergic reaction.

Yes   No   **2.** This victim is likely experiencing a type of shock known as anaphylaxis.

Yes   No   **3.** The condition this victim is experiencing is life threatening, and medical care is needed.

Yes   No   **4.** If the victim has a prescribed epinephrine auto-injector, help her use it.

Yes   No   **5.** Place this victim in the usual shock position—lying down with the legs raised.

Answers: **1.** Yes; **2.** Yes; **3.** Yes; **4.** Yes; **5.** No

▶ Check Your Knowledge

Directions: Circle Yes if you agree with the statement, and circle No if you disagree.

Yes   No   **1.** Raise the legs of *all* severely injured victims.

Yes   No   **2.** Prevent body heat loss by putting blankets under and over the victim.

Yes   No   **3.** A shock victim with possible spinal injuries should be placed in a seated position.

Yes   No   **4.** A shock victim with breathing difficulty or chest injury should be placed on his or her back with the legs raised.

Yes   No   **5.** Anxiety and restlessness are signs of shock.

Yes   No   **6.** An epinephrine auto-injector requires a doctor's prescription.

Yes   No   **7.** All severely injured or ill victims should be treated for shock.

Yes   No   **8.** Treat severely injured victims for shock even though there are no signs of it.

Yes   No   **9.** Anaphylaxis is a life-threatening breathing emergency.

Yes   No   **10.** Victims in shock have hot skin.

Answers: **1.** No; **2.** Yes; **3.** No; **4.** No; **5.** Yes; **6.** Yes; **7.** Yes; **8.** Yes; **9.** Yes; **10.** No

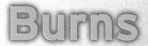

Burns

▶ Types of Burns

Burn injuries can be classified as thermal (heat), chemical, or electrical.

- *Thermal (heat) burns.* Thermal burns can be caused by flames, contact with hot objects, flammable vapor that ignites and causes a flash or an explosion, steam, or hot liquid.
- *Chemical burns.* Chemical agents can cause tissue damage and death if they come in contact with the skin. Three types of chemicals—acids, alkalis, and organic compounds—are responsible for most chemical burns.
- *Electrical burns.* The severity of injury from contact with electric current depends on the type of current (direct or alternating), the voltage, the area of the body exposed, and the duration of contact.

▶ Thermal Burns

Evaluate a thermal burn using the following steps. These steps form the basis for treatment of thermal burns.

1. Determine the depth (degree) of the burn. Historically, burns have been described as first-degree, second-degree, and third-degree injuries.

Medical care professionals use the terms *superficial, partial thickness,* and *full thickness* because they are more descriptive of the extent of tissue damage.

- <u>First-degree (superficial) burns</u> affect the skin's outer layer (epidermis) **Figure 6-1**. Characteristics include redness, mild swelling, tenderness, and pain. Sunburn is a common example of a first-degree burn. Healing occurs without scarring, usually within a week.
- <u>Second-degree (partial-thickness) burns</u> extend through the skin's entire outer layer and into the inner layer **Figure 6-2**. Blisters, swelling, weeping of fluids, and pain identify these burns. Intact blisters provide a sterile, waterproof covering. Once a blister breaks, a weeping wound results, and the risk of infection increases. Large second-degree burns require medical care.
- <u>Third-degree (full-thickness) burns</u> are severe burns that penetrate all the skin layers and the underlying fat and muscle **Figure 6-3**. The skin looks leathery, waxy, or pearly gray, and sometimes charred. The victim feels no pain from a third-degree burn because the nerve endings have been damaged or destroyed. Any pain felt is from surrounding burns of lesser degrees. A third-degree burn requires medical care.

2. Determine the extent of the burn. Part of deter-

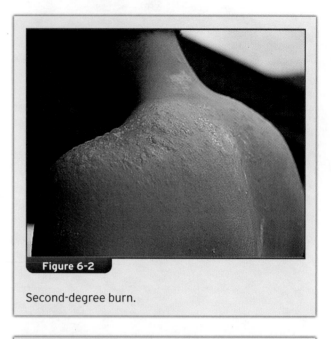

Figure 6-2

Second-degree burn.

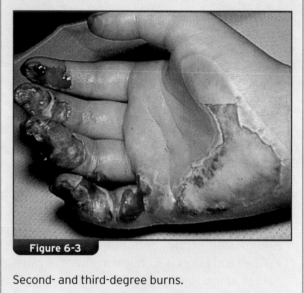

Figure 6-3

Second- and third-degree burns.

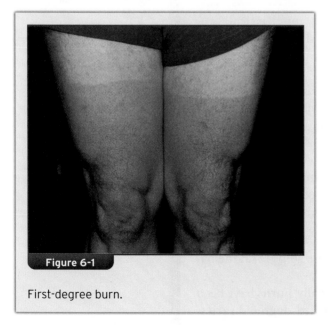

Figure 6-1

First-degree burn.

mining the severity of a burn requires you to estimate how much body surface area (BSA) the burn covers. You can use the Rule of the Palm to estimate the size of a burn. The victim's hand, excluding the fingers and the thumb, represents about 1% of his or her total body surface **Figure 6-4**.

3. Determine which parts of the body are burned. Burns on the face, hands, feet, and genitals are more severe than on other body parts.

4. Determine whether other injuries or preexisting medical problems are present or if the victim is elderly or very young. A medical problem or belonging to one of these age groups increases a burn's severity.

▶ Care for Thermal Burns

Burn care aims to reduce pain, protect against infection, and determine the need for medical care. Most burns are minor and can be managed without medical care. If clothing is burning, have the victim roll on the ground using the "stop, drop, and roll" method. Smother the flames with a blanket or douse the victim with water. Seek medical care if any of the following conditions apply:

- The victim is younger than 5 or older than 55 years.
- The victim has difficulty breathing.
- Other injuries exist.
- An electrical injury exists.
- The face, hands, feet, or genitals are burned.
- Child abuse is suspected.
- The surface area of a second-degree burn is larger than 20% of the victim's BSA.
- The burn is third degree.

Care for First-Degree Burns

1. Cool the burn with cold water until the part is pain free (at least 10 minutes) **Figure 6-5**.
2. After the burn cools, apply an aloe vera gel or

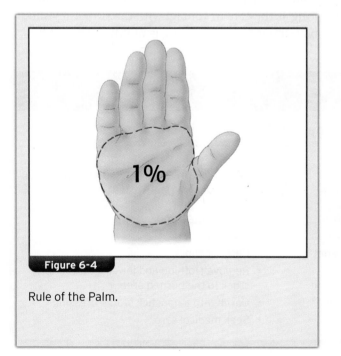

Figure 6-4

Rule of the Palm.

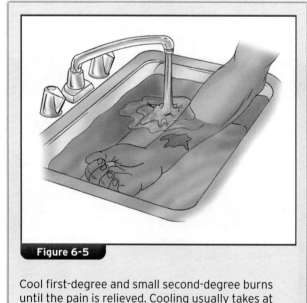

Figure 6-5

Cool first-degree and small second-degree burns until the pain is relieved. Cooling usually takes at least 10 minutes.

skin moisturizer to keep the skin moistened and to reduce itching and peeling.

3. If available, give ibuprofen to relieve pain and inflammation. Give acetaminophen to children.

Care for Small Second-Degree Burns (<20% BSA)

1. Remove clothing and jewelry from the burned area.
2. Cool the burn with cold water until the part is pain free (at least 10 minutes).
3. After the burn has been cooled, apply antibiotic ointment.
4. Cover the burn loosely with a dry, nonstick, sterile or clean dressing to keep the burn clean, prevent evaporative moisture loss, and reduce pain.
5. If available, give ibuprofen to relieve pain and inflammation. For children, give acetaminophen.

Care for Large Second-Degree (>20% BSA) and All Third-Degree Burns

1. Monitor breathing.
2. Remove clothing and jewelry that is not stuck to the burned area.
3. Cover the burn with a dry, nonstick, sterile or clean dressing.

CAUTION

DO NOT cool more than 20% of an adult's body surface area (10% for a child) except to extinguish flames. Widespread cooling can cause hypothermia.

DO NOT break any blisters. Intact blisters serve as excellent burn dressings. Cover a ruptured blister with an antibiotic ointment and a nonstick sterile or clean dressing.

DO NOT apply salve, ointment, grease, butter, cream, spray, a home remedy, or any other coating on a burn. Such coatings are not sterile and can lead to infection. The exception to this rule is after cooling a burn, aloe vera gel can be applied on a first-degree burn and an antibiotic ointment on small second-degree burns.

4. Care for shock.
5. Seek medical care.

▶ Chemical Burns

A chemical burn results when a caustic or corrosive substance touches the skin **Figure 6-6**. Examples of such substances include acids, alkalis, and organic compounds. Because chemicals continue to burn as long as they are in contact with the skin, they should be removed from the skin as rapidly as possible.

Thermal Burn Care

Degree of the Burn?

First-Degree (Superficial) Burn

- Cool the burned area until the pain stops.
- Apply aloe vera gel or other moisturizer.

Small Second-Degree (Partial-Thickness) Burn

- Remove clothing and jewelry from burned area.
- Cool the burned area until the pain stops.
- Apply antibiotic ointment and cover with a nonstick sterile dressing.

Large Second-Degree (Partial-Thickness) or Third-Degree (Full-Thickness) Burn

- Monitor breathing and provide care as needed.
- Care for shock.
- Remove clothing and jewelry that is not stuck to the burned area.
- Cover with a nonstick sterile dressing.
- Seek medical care.

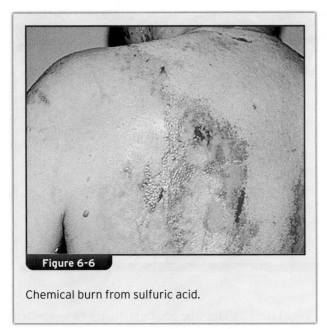

Figure 6-6

Chemical burn from sulfuric acid.

First aid is the same for most chemical burns, except for a few specific ones for which a chemical neutralizer has to be used. Alkalis such as drain cleaners cause more serious burns than acids such as battery acid because they penetrate deeper and remain active longer. Organic compounds such as petroleum products are also capable of burning.

CAUTION

DO NOT apply water under high pressure—it will drive the chemical deeper into the tissue.

Care for Chemical Burns

1. Immediately flush the area with a large quantity of water for 20 minutes Figure 6-7A, B . If the chemical is a dry powder, brush the powder from the skin before flushing Figure 6-8 .
2. Remove the victim's contaminated clothing and jewelry while flushing with water.
3. Cover the affected area with a dry, sterile or clean dressing.
4. Seek medical care.

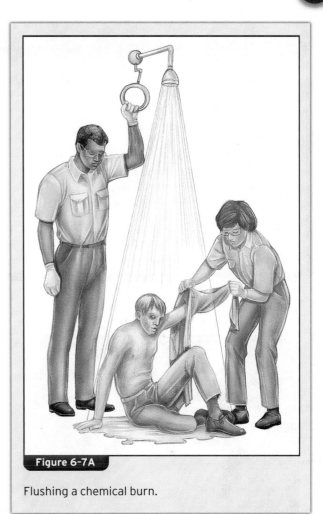

Figure 6-7A

Flushing a chemical burn.

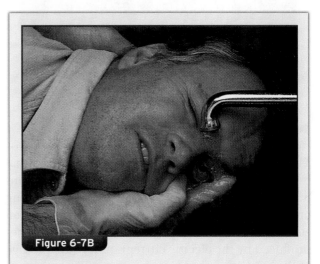

Figure 6-7B

Flush a chemical in an eye from the bridge of the nose outward.

Chemical Burns

Dry or Wet Chemical?

Dry

- Brush off chemical.
- Wash with water for 20 minutes.
- Remove clothing and jewelry.
- Do not try to neutralize.
- Seek medical care.

Wet

- Wash immediately with water for 20 minutes.
- Remove clothing and jewelry.
- Do not try to neutralize.
- Seek medical care.

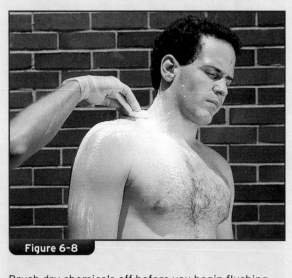

Figure 6-8

Brush dry chemicals off before you begin flushing.

▶ Electrical Burns

There are three types of electrical injuries: thermal burn (flame), arc burn (flash), and true electrical injury (contact). A thermal burn results when clothing or objects in contact with the skin are ignited by an electric current. These injuries are caused by the flames produced by the electric current, not by the passage of the electric current or arc.

An arc burn occurs when electricity jumps, or arcs, from one spot to another. Although the dura-tion of the flash may be brief, it usually causes extensive superficial injuries.

A true electrical injury happens when an electric current passes directly through the body, which can disrupt the normal heart rhythm and cause cardiac arrest, other internal injuries, and burns. Usually, the electricity exits where the body touches a surface or comes in contact with a ground (for example, a metal object). This type of injury is often characterized by an entrance and exit wound **Figure 6-9**.

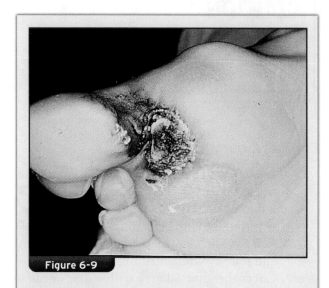

Figure 6-9

Electrical burn exit wound on toe.

Care for Electrical Burns

1. Make sure the area is safe. Unplug, disconnect, or turn off the power. If that is impossible, call 9-1-1.
2. Monitor breathing.
3. If the victim fell, check for a possible spinal injury.
4. Care for shock.
5. Call 9-1-1 for medical care.

Contact with a Power Line (Outdoors)

If the electrical shock is from contact with a downed power line, the power must be turned off before it is safe to approach a victim in contact with the wire. Do not attempt to move downed wires unless you are trained and equipped with tools that can handle the high voltage. Do not attempt to move any wires, even with wooden poles, tools with wood handles, or tree branches. Do not use objects with a high moisture content, and certainly not metal objects.

Contact Inside Buildings

Most electrical burns that occur indoors are caused by faulty electrical equipment or careless use of electrical appliances. Turn off the electricity at the circuit breaker, fuse box, or outside switch box, or unplug the appliance if the plug is undamaged. Do not touch the appliance or the victim until the current is off.

Meeting OSHA Guidelines

This chapter covers the following *OSHA Best Practices Guide: Fundamentals of a Workplace First Aid Program (2006)*:

5. Responding to Non-Life-Threatening Emergencies
   • Burns
     • Assessing the severity of a burn;
     • Recognizing whether a burn is thermal, electrical, or chemical and the appropriate first aid;
     • Reviewing corrosive chemicals at a specific worksite, along with appropriate first aid.

Electrical Burns

Victim Still in Contact with Electricity?

No Contact with Electricity

• If victim is motionless, open the airway, check breathing, and treat accordingly.
• Care for shock.
• Care for the electrical burn like you would a third-degree burn.
• Call 9-1-1.

Still in Contact with Electricity

• Turn off electricity at fuse box, circuit breaker, or outside fuse box, or unplug appliance.
• Call 9-1-1 if victim is in contact with downed power lines.

► Thermal (Heat) Burns

What to Look For	What to Do
First-degree burn • Redness • Mild swelling • Pain	1. Cool the burn with cold water. 2. Apply aloe vera gel or a skin moisturizer. 3. If available, give an over-the-counter pain medication.
Second-degree burn • Blisters • Swelling • Pain • Weeping of fluid	If burn is small (<20% BSA): 1. Cool the burn with cold water. 2. Apply antibiotic ointment. 3. Cover with a dry, nonstick, sterile dressing. 4. If available, give an over-the-counter pain medication. If burn is large (>20% BSA): 1. Follow steps for a third-degree burn.
Third-degree burns • Dry, leathery skin • Gray or charred skin	1. Monitor breathing and provide care as needed. 2. Cover burn with a dry, nonstick, sterile or clean dressing. 3. Care for shock. 4. Seek medical care.

► Chemical Burns

What to Look For	What to Do
• Stinging pain	1. Brush dry powder chemicals off skin. 2. Flush with a large amount of water for 20 minutes. 3. Remove victim's contaminated clothing and jewelry while flushing. 4. Cover area with a dry, sterile or clean dressing. 5. Seek medical care.

► Electrical Burns

What to Look For	What to Do
• Possible third-degree burn with entrance and exit wounds	1. Safety first! Unplug, disconnect, or turn off the electricity. 2. Open the airway, check breathing, and provide care as needed. 3. Care for burns as you would a third-degree burn. 4. Call 9-1-1.

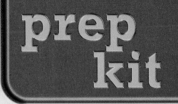
prep kit

▶ Key Terms

<u>first-degree (superficial) burn</u> A superficial burn that affects the skin's outer layer.

<u>second-degree (partial-thickness) burn</u> A partial-thickness burn that extends through the skin's entire outer layer and into the inner layer.

<u>third-degree (full-thickness) burn</u> A full-thickness burn that penetrates all the skin layers into the underlying fat and muscle.

▶ Assessment in Action

At a fast-food restaurant, a worker is burned on his forearm after bumping into a hot pan on the stove. The burned area is about the width of a tennis ball. Blisters are forming and the worker complains about the pain.

Directions: Circle Yes if you agree with the statement, and circle No if you disagree.

Yes No **1.** The size of the burn is probably about 1% of the worker's body surface area.

Yes No **2.** The blisters and pain are signs that the burn is a third-degree burn.

Yes No **3.** Reduce the pain and damage by running cold water over the burned area.

Yes No **4.** An antibiotic ointment can be applied to this burn only after cooling the area.

Yes No **5.** This victim needs medical care.

Answers: **1.** Yes; **2.** No; **3.** Yes; **4.** Yes; **5.** No

▶ Check Your Knowledge

Directions: Circle Yes if you agree with the statement, and circle No if you disagree.

Yes No **1.** The hands and feet are especially sensitive to being burned.

Yes No **2.** Petroleum jelly can be applied over a burn.

Yes No **3.** The Rule of the Palm determines the size of a burned area.

Yes No **4.** Neutralize an acid on the skin by using baking soda.

Yes No **5.** Use a large amount of water to flush chemicals off the body.

Yes No **6.** Brush a dry chemical off the skin before flushing with water.

Yes No **7.** When someone gets electrocuted, there can be two burn wounds: entrance and exit.

Yes No **8.** When a victim is in contact with a power line, use a tree branch to remove the wires.

Yes No **9.** Ibuprofen helps relieve pain and swelling.

Yes No **10.** Cold water can be used on any burn of any size.

Answers: **1.** Yes; **2.** No; **3.** Yes; **4.** No; **5.** Yes; **6.** Yes; **7.** Yes; **8.** No; **9.** Yes; **10.** No

Head and Spinal Injuries

Head Injuries

Any head injury is potentially serious. If not properly treated, injuries that seem minor could become life threatening. Head injuries include scalp wounds, skull fractures, and brain injuries. Spinal injuries (that is, neck and back injuries) can also be present in head-injured victims.

▶ Scalp Wounds

The scalp has many blood vessels, so any cut can cause heavy bleeding. A bleeding scalp wound does not affect the blood supply to the brain.

Care for Scalp Wounds

To care for a scalp wound:
1. Apply a sterile or clean dressing and direct pressure to control bleeding **Figure 7-1**.
2. Keep the victim's head and shoulders slightly elevated to help control bleeding if no spinal injury is suspected.
3. Seek medical care.

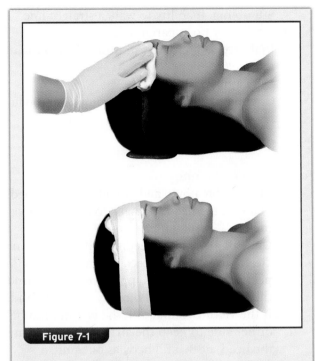

Figure 7-1

Apply direct pressure with a dry, sterile dressing to control bleeding.

▶ Skull Fracture

Significant force applied to the head may cause a <u>skull fracture</u>. This occurs when part of the skull (the bones forming the head) is broken.

Recognizing Skull Fracture

Signs of skull fracture include the following:

- Pain at the point of injury
- Deformity of the skull
- Drainage of clear or bloody fluid from the ears or nose
- Bruising under the eyes or behind an ear appearing several hours after the injury
- Changes in pupils (unequal, not reactive to light)
- Heavy scalp bleeding (A scalp wound may expose the skull or brain tissue.)
- Penetrating wound, such as from a bullet or an impaled object

Care for Skull Fracture

To care for a skull fracture:

1. Monitor breathing and provide care if needed.
2. Control any bleeding by applying a sterile or clean dressing and applying pressure around the edges of the wound, not directly on it **Figure 7-2** .
3. Stabilize the head and neck to prevent movement.
4. Seek medical care.

FYI

Head Injury Follow-up

Seek medical care if any of the following signs appear within 48 hours of a head injury. These symptoms are caused by excessive pressure on the brain.

- *Headache:* Severe headache, or one that lasts more than 1 or 2 days or gets worse
- *Nausea, vomiting:* Nausea that does not go away, or vomiting more than once
- *Drowsiness and confusion*
- *Vision and eye problems:* Double vision, eyes that do not move together, one pupil that appears larger than the other, or dilated pupils (larger than normal)
- *Mobility:* Weakness, numbness in arms or legs, or trouble walking
- *Speech:* Slurred speech or inability to talk
- *Seizures (convulsions)*

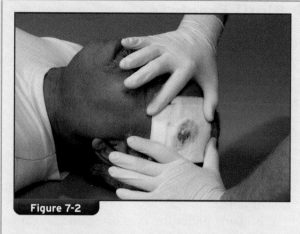

Figure 7-2

Apply pressure around the edges of the wound to control bleeding from a suspected skull fracture.

▶ Brain Injuries

The brain can be shaken by a blow to the head. A temporary disturbance of brain activity known as a <u>concussion</u> can result. Most concussions are mild, and people recover fully, but this process takes time. Concussions do not involve bleeding under the skull or swelling of brain tissue.

Recognizing Brain Injury

Signs of brain injury include the following:

- Befuddled facial expression (vacant stare)
- Slowness in answering questions
- Unawareness of where they are or day of week
- Slurred speech
- Stumbling, inability to walk a straight line
- Crying for no apparent reason
- Inability to recite the months of the year in reverse order
- Unresponsiveness
- Complaints of headache, dizziness, and nausea within minutes or hours of injury

Care for Brain Injuries

To care for a brain injury:

1. Monitor breathing and provide care if needed.
2. Stabilize the head and neck to prevent movement.
3. Control any scalp bleeding with a sterile or clean dressing and direct pressure. If you suspect a skull fracture, apply pressure around the wound edges, not directly on the wound.
4. If the victim vomits, roll the victim onto his or her side to keep the airway clear, moving the head, neck, and body as one unit.
5. Seek medical care.

CAUTION

DO NOT stop the flow of fluid from the ears or nose. Blocking the flow of either could increase pressure inside the skull.

DO NOT elevate the legs—that might increase pressure on the brain.

DO NOT clean an open skull injury—infection of the brain may result.

Head Injuries

Type of Injury?

Scalp Wound

- Apply sterile or clean dressing and direct pressure.
- Slightly elevate the victim's head and shoulders if no spinal injury is suspected.
- Seek medical care.

Skull Fracture or Brain Injury

- Monitor breathing and provide care if needed.
- Consider possible spinal injury. Stabilize the victim's head and neck to prevent movement.
- Apply sterile or clean dressing; apply pressure around the edges of any wound, not directly on it.
- Seek medical care.

Eye Injuries

Eye injuries are common, particularly in sports. An eye injury can produce severe lifelong complications, including blindness. When in doubt about an injury's severity, seek medical care.

▶ Foreign Objects in Eye

Many different types of objects can enter the eye and cause significant damage. Even a small foreign object, such as a grain of sand, can produce severe irritation.

Care for Loose Foreign Objects in Eye

Try one or more of the following techniques to remove the object **Figure 7-3**.

1. Lift the upper lid over the lower lid, so that the lower lashes can brush the object off the inside of the upper lid. Have the victim blink a few times.
2. Hold the eyelid open, and gently rinse with warm water.
3. Examine the lower lid by pulling it down gently. If you can see the object, remove it with moistened sterile gauze or a clean cloth.
4. Examine the underside of the upper lid by grasping the lashes of the upper lid and rolling the lid upward over a stick or swab. If you can

see the object, remove it with moistened sterile gauze or a clean cloth.

CAUTION

DO NOT allow the victim to rub the eye.
DO NOT try to remove an embedded foreign object.
DO NOT use dry cotton (cotton balls or cotton-tipped swabs) or instruments such as tweezers to remove an object from an eye.

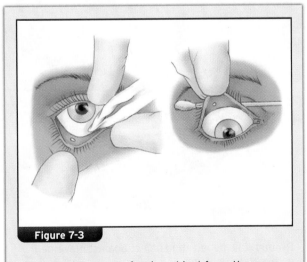

Figure 7-3

Locate and remove a foreign object from the eye.

▶ Penetrating Eye Injuries

Penetrating eye injuries result when a sharp object penetrates the eyeball and then is withdrawn or when an object remains embedded in the eye.

Care for Penetrating Eye Injuries

To care for a penetrating eye injury:

1. Stabilize long embedded objects with bulky dressings or clean cloths held in place **Figure 7-4** .
2. Have the victim keep the uninjured eye closed.
3. Call 9-1-1.

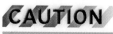

DO NOT wash the eye out with water.
DO NOT try to remove an object stuck in the eye.
DO NOT press on an injured eyeball or penetrating object.

▶ Blows to the Eye

Blows to the eye range from an ordinary black eye to severe damage that threatens eyesight **Figure 7-5** .

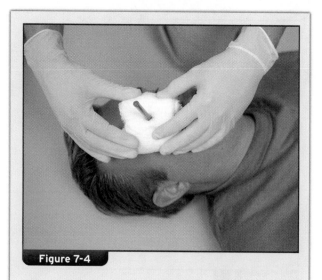

Figure 7-4

Protecting a penetrating object against movement with a bulky dressing.

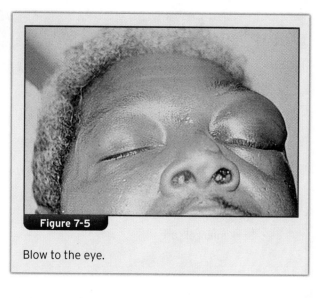

Figure 7-5

Blow to the eye.

Care for Blows to the Eye

To care for a blow to the eye:

1. Apply an ice or cold pack for about 15 minutes to reduce pain and swelling. Do not apply it directly on the eyeball or apply any pressure on the eye.
2. Seek medical care if there is pain, double vision, or reduced vision.

▶ Eye Avulsion

An <u>eye avulsion</u> occurs from a blow to the eye that knocks the eyeball from its socket.

Care for Eye Avulsion

To care for an eye avulsion:

1. Cover the injured eye loosely with a sterile or clean moistened dressing. Do not try to push the eyeball back into the socket.
2. Protect the injured eye with a paper cup, held in place by tape.
3. Have the victim keep the uninjured eye closed.
4. Call 9-1-1.

▶ Cuts of the Eye or Lid

Cuts of the eye or lid require very careful repair to restore appearance and function **Figure 7-6** .

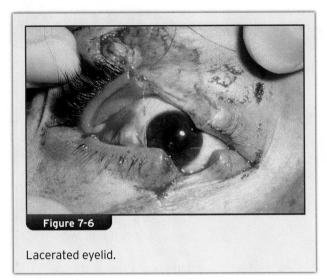

Figure 7-6

Lacerated eyelid.

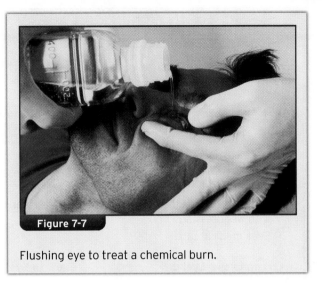

Figure 7-7

Flushing eye to treat a chemical burn.

Care for Cuts of the Eye or Lid

To care for a cut of the eye or lid:

1. If the eyeball is cut, do not apply pressure on it. If only the eyelid is cut, apply a sterile or clean dressing with gentle pressure.
2. Have the victim keep the uninjured eye closed.
3. Call 9-1-1.

▶ Chemicals in the Eye

Chemical burns of the eye, usually caused by an acid or alkaline solution, need immediate care because damage can occur in as little as 1 minute. They may cause the loss of vision.

Care for Chemicals in the Eye

To care for a chemical in the eye:

1. Hold the eye wide open and flush with warm water for at least 20 minutes, continuously and gently **Figure 7-7**. Irrigate from the nose side of the eye toward the outside to avoid flushing material into the other eye.

2. Loosely bandage the eyes with wet dressings.
3. Seek medical care.

CAUTION

DO NOT try to neutralize the chemical. Water usually is readily available and is better for eye irrigation.

DO NOT bandage the eye tightly.

▶ Eye Burns from Light

Burns can result from looking at a source of ultraviolet light, such as a welder's arc or the glare off bright snow. Severe pain occurs several hours after exposure.

Care for Eye Burns from Light

To care for an eye burn from light:

1. Cover both eyes with wet dressings and cold packs. Tell the victim not to rub the eyes.
2. Seek medical care.

Eye Injuries

Type of Eye Injury?

Chemical in Eye

- Hold eye open and flush with warm water for 20 minutes.
- Loosely bandage the eyes with wet dressings.
- Seek medical care.

Penetrating Eye Injury

- Stabilize a long object with bulky dressings and hold in place.
- Keep uninjured eye closed.
- Call 9-1-1.

Loose Object in Eye

- Pull upper eyelid down and over lower lid.
- Pull lower lid down and look at inner surface while victim looks up. If the object is seen, remove it with wet gauze.
- Lift upper eyelid. If the object is seen, remove it with wet gauze.

Cut on Eye or Eyelid

- If eyeball is cut, do not apply pressure.
- If only eyelid is cut, apply dressing with gentle pressure.
- Call 9-1-1.

Blow to Eye

- Apply an ice or cold pack for 15 minutes.
- Seek medical care if there is pain or double or reduced vision.

Nose Injuries

The nose often gets hit during sports activities, physical assaults, and motor vehicle crashes.

▶ Nosebleeds

Rupture of tiny blood vessels inside the nostrils by a blow to the nose, sneezing, or picking or blowing the nose causes most nosebleeds.

There are two types of nosebleeds:

- <u>Anterior nosebleeds</u> (*front of nose*) are the most common type of nosebleed (90%) and are normally easily cared for.
- A <u>posterior nosebleed</u> (*back of nose*) involves massive bleeding backward into the mouth or down the back of the throat. A posterior nosebleed is serious and requires medical care.

Care for Nosebleeds

To care for a nosebleed:

1. Place the victim in a seated position with the victim's head tilted slightly forward.
2. Pinch (or have the victim pinch) the soft parts of the nose between the thumb and two fingers with steady pressure for 5 to 10 minutes **Figure 7-8**.
3. Seek medical care if any of the following applies:
   - Bleeding cannot be controlled.
   - You suspect a posterior nosebleed.
   - The victim has high blood pressure or is taking anticoagulants (blood thinners) or large doses of aspirin.
   - Bleeding occurs after a blow to the nose, and you suspect a broken nose.

CAUTION

DO NOT allow the victim to tilt his or her head backward.

DO NOT probe the nose with a cotton-tipped swab.

DO NOT move the victim's head and neck if a spinal injury is suspected.

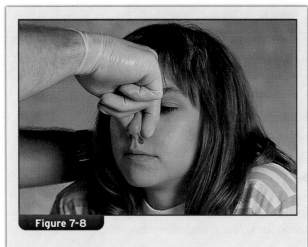

Figure 7-8

Control bleeding from the nose by pinching the nostrils together.

▶ Broken Nose

A blow to the nose can break the nose.

Recognizing a Broken Nose

The signs of a broken nose include the following:
- Pain, swelling, and possibly crooked nose
- Bleeding and breathing difficulty through the nostrils
- Black eyes appearing 1 to 2 days after the injury

Care for a Broken Nose

To care for a broken nose:
1. If bleeding, provide care as for a nosebleed.
2. Apply an ice or cold pack to the nose for 15 minutes. Do not try to straighten a crooked nose.
3. Seek medical care.

Mouth Injuries

Mouth injuries can involve damage to the lips, tongue, and teeth. These injuries can cause considerable pain and anxiety.

▶ Bitten Lip or Tongue

Care for Bitten Lip or Tongue

To care for a bitten lip or tongue:
1. Apply direct pressure.
2. Apply an ice or cold pack.
3. If the bleeding does not stop, seek medical care.

▶ Knocked-Out Tooth

A knocked-out tooth is a dental emergency **Figure 7-9**. You have about 30 minutes to reach a dentist for successful replantation of the tooth, so it is important to locate the tooth and prevent it from becoming dried out, and to protect the ligament fibers on the roots from damage.

Care for a Knocked-Out Tooth

To care for a knocked-out tooth:
1. Have the victim rinse his or her mouth, and place a rolled gauze pad in the socket to control bleeding.
2. Find the tooth and handle it by the crown, not the root.
3. Get the victim to a dentist promptly so the tooth can be successfully replaced in its socket. If more serious injuries exist, seek medical care.

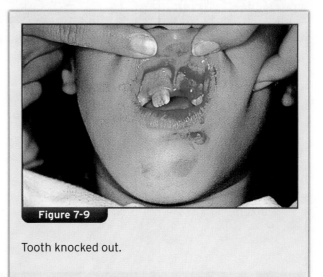

Figure 7-9

Tooth knocked out.

4. The tooth should be kept moist. Several options exist:
   - If the victim is an adult and alert, the tooth can be laid inside the lower lip, between the teeth and lip.
   - If it is not possible to place the tooth in the mouth, have the victim spit into a cup, and place the tooth in the saliva.
   - If neither of the preceding options is possible, the tooth can be placed in cool milk. DO NOT place it in water.

FYI

Dental Emergencies

Broken Tooth

Rinse the mouth with warm water. Apply a cold pack to the outside of the cheek. Contact a dentist.

Objects Caught Between Teeth

Try to gently remove the object with dental floss. If the object cannot be dislodged, contact a dentist.

Toothache

Rinse the mouth with warm water. Gently use dental floss to remove any debris caught between the teeth. If the pain persists, contact a dentist.

FYI

Reinserting a Knocked-Out Tooth

If you are in a remote area more than 1 hour away from definitive medical or dental care, you could rinse the tooth lightly and attempt to reinsert it.

▶ Toothache

Toothaches can be extremely painful and cause headaches, fever, and sleeplessness.

Care for Toothaches

To care for toothaches:

1. Rinse the mouth with warm water to clean it out.
2. Use dental floss to remove any food that might be trapped between the teeth.
3. Give the victim pain medication (aspirin, acetaminophen, or ibuprofen). Do not place medication on gums.
4. Seek dental care.

Mouth Injuries

Type of Injury?

Bitten Lip or Tongue	Toothache	Tooth Knocked Out	Broken Tooth
• Apply direct pressure. • Apply an ice or cold pack. • If the bleeding does not stop, seek medical care.	• Rinse mouth with warm water. • Remove any trapped food with dental floss. • See a dentist.	• Rinse mouth with water. • Control bleeding. • Preserve the tooth in the victim's saliva or milk. • Take tooth and victim to a dentist.	• Rinse mouth with warm water. • Apply an ice or cold pack on outside of cheek. • See a dentist.

Spinal Injuries

Motor vehicle crashes, direct blows, falls from heights, physical assaults, and sports injuries are common causes of spinal injury. Suspect spine injuries in victims with significant head injuries, since the two are often associated.

Recognizing Spinal Injuries

The signs of spinal injuries include the following:

- Inability to move arms and/or legs
- Numbness, tingling, weakness, or burning sensation in the arms and/or legs
- Deformity (odd-looking angle of the victim's head and neck)
- Neck or back pain

Care for Spinal Injuries

To care for a spinal injury:

1. Stabilize the head and neck to prevent movement **Figure 7-10** .
2. If unresponsive, open the airway, check breathing, and provide any needed care.
3. Call 9-1-1.

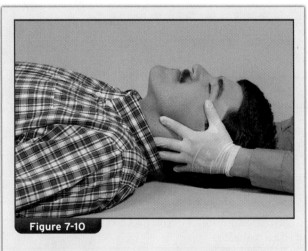

Figure 7-10

Prevent movement of the head and neck.

Meeting OSHA Guidelines

This chapter covers the following *OSHA Best Practices Guide: Fundamentals of a Workplace First Aid Program (2006)*:

5. Responding to Non-Life-Threatening Emergencies
   - Musculoskeletal Injuries
     - Head, neck, back and spinal injuries
   - Eye Injuries
     - First aid for eye injuries;
     - First aid for chemical burns.
   - Mouth and Teeth Injuries
     - Oral injuries; lip and tongue injuries; broken and missing teeth;
     - The importance of preventing aspiration of blood and/or teeth.

▶ Head Injuries

What to Look For | What to Do

Scalp wound

1. Apply a sterile or clean dressing and direct pressure to control bleeding.
2. Keep head and shoulders raised.
3. Seek medical care.

Skull fracture
- Pain at point of injury
- Deformity of the skull
- Clear or bloody fluid draining from ears or nose
- Bruising under eyes or behind an ear
- Changes in pupils
- Heavy scalp bleeding
- Penetrating wound

1. Monitor breathing and provide care if needed.
2. Control bleeding by applying pressure around the edges of wound.
3. Stabilize the victim's head and neck against movement.
4. Seek medical care.

Brain injury (concussion)
- Befuddled facial expression (vacant stare)
- Slownesss in answering questions
- Unawareness of where they are or day of week
- Slurred speech
- Stumbling, inability to walk a straight line
- Crying for no apparent reason
- Inability to recite months of year in reverse order
- Unresponsiveness
- Headache, dizziness, and nausea

1. Monitor breathing and provide care if needed.
2. Stabilize the victim's head and neck against movement.
3. Control any scalp bleeding.
4. Seek medical care.

▶ Eye Injuries

What to Look For | What to Do

Loose foreign object in eye

1. Look for object underneath both lids.
2. If seen, remove with wet gauze.

Penetrating eye injury

1. If object is still in eye, protect eye and stabilize long objects.
2. Call 9-1-1.

Blow to the eye

1. Apply an ice or cold pack. DO NOT place ice or cold pack on eyeball.
2. Seek medical care if vision is affected.

Eye avulsion
- Eyeball knocked out of its socket

1. Cover eye loosely with wet dressing.
2. DO NOT try to put eye back into socket.
3. Call 9-1-1.

Cuts of eye or lid

1. If eyeball is cut, DO NOT apply pressure.
2. If only eyelid is cut, apply dressing with gentle pressure.
3. Call 9-1-1.

Chemicals in eye	1. Flush with warm water for 20 minutes and loosely bandage with wet dressings. 2. Seek medical care.
Eye burns from light	1. Cover eyes with cold, wet dressings. 2. Seek medical care.

▶ Nose Injuries

What to Look For	What to Do

Nosebleeds	1. Keep victim sitting up with head level or tilted forward slightly.
	2. Pinch soft parts of nose for 5 to 10 minutes.
	3. Seek medical care if:
	  • Bleeding does not stop
	  • Blood is going down throat
	  • Bleeding is associated with a broken nose

Broken nose • Pain, swelling, and possibly crooked nose • Bleeding and breathing difficulty through nostrils • Black eyes appearing 1 to 2 days after injury	1. Care for nosebleed. 2. Apply an ice or cold pack for 15 minutes. 3. Seek medical care.

▶ Mouth Injuries

What to Look For	What to Do
Bitten lip or tongue	1. Apply direct pressure. 2. Apply an ice or cold pack.
Knocked-out tooth	1. Control bleeding (place rolled gauze in socket). 2. Find tooth and preserve it in milk or the victim's saliva. Handle the tooth by the crown, not the root. 3. See dentist as soon as possible.
Toothache	1. Rinse mouth and use dental floss to removed trapped food. 2. Give pain medication. 3. Seek dental care.

▶ Spinal Injuries

What to Look For	What to Do
• Inability to move arms and/or legs • Numbness, tingling, weakness, or burning feeling in arms and/or legs • Deformity (head and neck at an odd angle) • Neck or back pain	1. Stabilize the head and neck against movement. 2. If unresponsive, open the victim's airway and check breathing. 3. Call 9-1-1.

prep kit

▶ Key Terms

<u>anterior nosebleed</u> Bleeding from the front of the nose.

<u>concussion</u> A temporary disturbance of brain activity caused by a blow to the head.

<u>eye avulsion</u> Forcible separation of the eyeball from its socket.

<u>posterior nosebleed</u> Bleeding from the back of the nose into the mouth or down the back of the throat.

<u>skull fracture</u> A break of part of the skull (head bones).

▶ Assessment in Action

You see a middle-aged man walking down the street; suddenly, he is struck by a piece of wood that has fallen 50 feet from a construction site above. The victim collapses and remains on the ground. He is slow to answer questions and cannot remember where he is or the day of the week. He says he feels lightheaded and nauseated. You see a lot of blood coming from a wound on his head.

Directions: Circle Yes if you agree with the statement, and circle No if you disagree.

Yes   No   1. Head-injured victims should be checked for possible spinal injury.

Yes   No   2. You think the victim may have suffered a skull fracture, so you press around the wound's edges rather than applying hard pressure over the wound to control the bleeding.

Yes   No   3. To treat for shock, this victim should be placed flat on his back with his legs elevated.

Yes   No   4. You do not suspect a concussion because the victim is still alert.

Yes   No   5. Minimize head and neck movement by not touching the victim—leave him as you found him.

Answers: 1. Yes; 2. Yes; 3. No; 4. No; 5. Yes

▶ Check Your Knowledge

Directions: Circle Yes if you agree with the statement, and circle No if you disagree.

Yes   No   1. Remove objects embedded in an eyeball.

Yes   No   2. Scalp wounds have very little bleeding.

Yes   No   3. Scrub and rinse the roots of a knocked-out tooth.

Yes   No   4. After a blow to the area around an eye, apply a cold pack.

Yes   No   5. Tears are sufficient to flush a chemical from the eye.

Yes   No   6. Use clean, damp gauze to remove an object from the eyelid's surface.

Yes   No   7. Preserve a knocked-out tooth in mouthwash.

Yes   No   8. Do not move a victim with a suspected spinal injury.

Yes   No   9. Inability to move the hands or feet, or both, may indicate a spinal injury.

Yes   No   10. To care for a nosebleed, have the injured person sit down and tilt his or her head back.

Answers: 1. No; 2. No; 3. No; 4. Yes; 5. No; 6. Yes; 7. No; 8. Yes; 9. Yes; 10. No

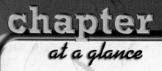

Chest, Abdominal, and Pelvic Injuries

▶ Chest Injuries

Chest injuries can be closed or open. In a <u>closed chest injury</u>, the victim's skin is not broken. This type of injury is usually caused by blunt trauma. In an <u>open chest injury</u>, the skin has been broken and the chest wall is penetrated by an object such as a knife or bullet.

A responsive chest injury victim should usually sit up or, if the injury is on a side, be placed with the injured side down. This position prevents blood inside the chest cavity from seeping into the uninjured side and allows the uninjured side to expand.

Recognizing Rib Fractures

Rib fractures are a closed chest injury. The most common type of rib fracture is ribs fractured by a blow or a fall. A <u>flail chest</u> results when several ribs in the same area are broken in more than one place. The care for an isolated rib fracture and for flail chest is the same.

The signs of a rib fracture include:
- Sharp pain, especially when victim takes a deep breath, coughs, or moves
- Shallow breathing
- Victim holds the injured area, trying to reduce pain

Care for Rib Fractures

To care for a rib fracture:
1. Help the victim find the most comfortable resting position.
2. Stabilize the ribs by having the victim hold a pillow or other similar soft object against the injured area, or use bandages to hold the pillow in place **Figure 8-1** .
3. Seek medical care.

Recognizing an Embedded (Impaled) Object

Embedded (impaled) objects are open chest injuries. The sign of an embedded (impaled object) is:
- Object stuck in the chest, such as a knife

Care for an Embedded (Impaled) Object

To care for an embedded (impaled) object:
1. DO NOT remove object. Removing an embedded object can cause more damage.
2. Use bulky dressings or cloth to stabilize the object.
3. Call 9-1-1.

Recognizing a Sucking Chest Wound

A sucking chest wound results when a chest wound allows air to pass into and out of the chest cavity with each breath.
The signs of a sucking chest wound include:
- Blood bubbling out of a chest wound
- Sound of air being sucked into and out of the chest wound

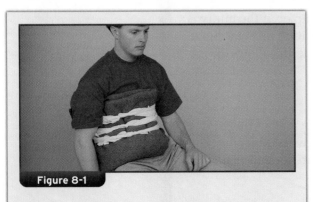

Figure 8-1

Stabilize chest with a soft object, such as a pillow, coat, or blanket (hold or tie).

Care for a Sucking Chest Wound

To care for a sucking chest wound:
1. Seal the wound with plastic or aluminum foil to stop air from entering the chest cavity. Tape three sides of the plastic or foil in place **Figure 8-2** . If neither item is available, you can use your gloved hand. This treatment prevents air from entering the chest but allows air to escape.
2. If the victim has trouble breathing or seems to be getting worse, remove the cover (or your hand) to let air escape, and then reapply.
3. Lay victim on injured side.
4. Call 9-1-1.

▶ Abdominal Injuries

Abdominal injuries are either open or closed. Closed abdominal injuries occur as the result of a direct blow from a blunt object. Open abdominal injuries include penetrating wounds, embedded (impaled) objects, and protruding organs. The risk of infection is high. An embedded (impaled) object in the abdomen is cared for in the same manner as an embedded object in the chest: Stabilize the object and call 9-1-1.

Recognizing a Closed Abdominal Injury

Look for bruises or other marks on the abdomen that indicate blunt injury. Examine the abdomen by gently pressing with your fingertips. Observe for pain, tenderness, muscle tightness, and rigidity. A normal abdomen is soft and not tender when pressed.

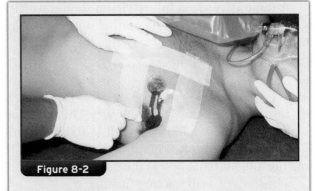

Figure 8-2

For a sucking chest wound, tape three sides of the plastic or foil in place.

Chest, Abdominal, and Pelvic Injuries

Injured Area?

Chest Injury

- If a sucking chest wound exists, cover with plastic or foil and tape down on three sides.
- If possible rib fracture exists, stabilize the ribs and chest.
- Do not remove impaled object; stabilize long object with bulky dressings.
- Call 9-1-1.

Abdominal Injury

- If organs are protruding, cover with moist, sterile or clean dressings.
- Do not remove impaled object; stabilize long object with bulky dressings.
- Call 9-1-1.

Pelvic Injury

- Keep the victim still.
- Care for shock.
- Call 9-1-1.

The signs of a closed abdominal injury include:
- Bruises or other marks
- Pain, tenderness, muscle tightness, and rigidity observed while gently pressing with your fingertips on the abdomen

Care for a Closed Abdominal Injury

To care for a closed abdominal injury:
1. Place the victim in a comfortable position with the legs pulled up toward the abdomen.
2. Care for shock.
3. Seek medical care.

Recognizing a Protruding Organ

A <u>protruding organ injury</u> refers to a severe injury to the abdomen in which the internal organs escape or protrude from the wound.

Care for a Protruding Organ

To care for protruding organs:
1. Place the victim in a comfortable position with the legs pulled up toward the abdomen.
2. Cover protruding organs loosely with a moist, sterile or clean dressing **Figures 8-3A, B**.

3. Care for shock.
4. Call 9-1-1.

▶ Pelvic Injuries

Injuries to the pelvis are usually caused by a motor vehicle crash or a fall from a height. Pelvic fractures can be life threatening because of the large amount of blood that could be lost if the femoral artery is damaged.

Recognizing Pelvic Fractures

The signs of a pelvic injury include:
- Pain in the hip, groin, or back that increases with movement
- Inability to walk or stand
- Signs of shock

Care for Pelvic Fractures

To care for a pelvic injury:
1. Keep the victim still.
2. Care for shock.
3. Call 9-1-1.

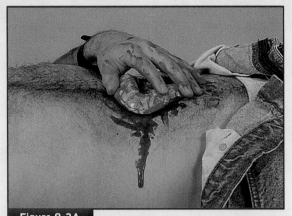

Figure 8-3A

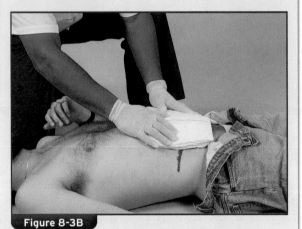

Figure 8-3B

Bandaging an open abdominal wound. **A.** Open abdominal wounds are serious injuries. **B.** Cover organs with a moist, sterile or clean dressing.

CAUTION

DO NOT try to reinsert protruding organs into the abdomen—you could introduce infection or damage the organs.

DO NOT cover the organs tightly.

DO NOT cover the organs with any material that clings or disintegrates when wet.

DO NOT give the victim anything to eat or drink.

Meeting OSHA Guidelines

This chapter covers the following *OSHA Best Practices Guide: Fundamentals of a Workplace First Aid Program (2006)*:

4. Responding to Life-Threatening Emergencies
   • Responding to Medical Emergencies
     • Chest pain;
     • Abdominal injury;
     • Impaled object

▶ Chest Injuries

What to Look For

Rib fractures
- Sharp pain with deep breaths, coughing, or moving
- Shallow breathing
- Holding of injured area to reduce pain

What to Do

1. Place victim in comfortable position.
2. Support ribs with a pillow, blanket, or coat (either holding or tying with bandages).
3. Seek medical care.

Embedded (impaled) object
- Object remains in wound

1. DO NOT remove object from wound.
2. Use bulky dressings or cloths to stabilize the object.
3. Call 9-1-1.

Sucking chest wound
- Blood bubbling out of wound
- Sound of air being sucked in and out of wound

1. Seal wound to stop air from entering chest; tape three sides of plastic or use gloved hand.
2. Remove cover to let air escape if victim worsens or has trouble breathing.
3. Call 9-1-1.

▶ Abdominal Injuries

What to Look For

Blow to abdomen (closed)
- Bruise or other marks
- Muscle tightness and rigidity felt while gently pushing on abdomen

What to Do

1. Place victim in comfortable position with legs pulled up toward the abdomen.
2. Care for shock.
3. Seek medical care.

Protruding organs (open)
- Internal organs escaping from abdominal wound

1. Place victim in a comfortable position with the legs pulled up toward the abdomen.
2. DO NOT reinsert organs into the abdomen.
3. Cover organs with a moist, sterile or clean dressing.
4. Care for shock.
5. Call 9-1-1.

▶ Pelvic Injuries

What to Look For

Pelvic fractures
- Pain in hip, groin, or back that increases with movement
- Inability to walk or stand
- Signs of shock

What to Do

1. Keep victim still.
2. Care for shock.
3. Call 9-1-1.

prep kit

▶ Key Terms

closed abdominal injuries Injuries to the abdomen that occur as a result of a direct blow from a blunt object.

closed chest injury An injury to the chest in which the skin is not broken; usually due to blunt trauma.

flail chest A condition that occurs when several ribs in the same area are broken in more than one place.

open abdominal injuries Injuries to the abdomen that include penetrating wounds and protruding organs.

open chest injury An injury to the chest in which the chest wall itself is penetrated, either by a fractured rib or, more frequently, by an external object such as a bullet or knife.

protruding organ injury A severe injury to the abdomen in which the internal organs escape or protrude from the wound.

sucking chest wound A chest wound that allows air to pass into and out of the chest cavity with each breath.

▶ Assessment in Action

A 45-year-old repairman falls while carrying replacement glass for a broken window. The new glass breaks into several jagged pieces. You find the repairman lying on his back with a blood-soaked shirt. You see a lacerated abdomen with several loops of intestine protruding from the laceration.

Directions: Circle Yes if you agree with the statement, and circle No if you disagree.

Yes   No   1. Gently push the protruding intestine back into the wound.

Yes   No   2. Place a moist dressing over the protruding intestine.

Yes   No   3. Place the victim on his back with the knees bent.

Yes   No   4. Cover the victim with a blanket or coat.

Yes   No   5. Give the victim something to drink.

Answers: 1. No; 2. Yes; 3. Yes; 4. Yes; 5. No

▶ Check Your Knowledge

Directions: Circle Yes if you agree with the statement, and circle No if you disagree.

Yes   No   1. Stabilize a broken rib with a soft object such as a pillow or blanket tied to the chest.

Yes   No   2. Cover a sucking chest wound with a piece of plastic taped down on three sides.

Yes   No   3. Remove a penetrating or impaled object from the chest or the abdomen.

Yes   No   4. A flail chest refers to a single broken rib.

Yes   No   5. Keep the victim with a broken pelvis still.

Yes   No   6. Sharp pain while breathing can be a sign of a rib fracture.

Yes   No   7. Rib fractures should be treated by tightly taping the chest.

Yes   No   8. Most victims with abdominal injuries are more comfortable with their knees bent.

Yes   No   9. Leave a chest wound alone if you hear air being sucked in and out.

Yes   No   10. A broken pelvis can threaten life because of the large amount of blood lost.

Answers: 1. Yes; 2. Yes; 3. No; 4. No; 5. Yes; 6. Yes; 7. No; 8. Yes; 9. No; 10. Yes

Bone, Joint, and Muscle Injuries

▶ Bone Injuries

The terms *broken bone* and <u>fracture</u> have the same meaning: a break or crack in a bone. There are two categories of fractures (Figure 9-1):

- <u>Closed fracture:</u> No open wound exists around the fracture site (Figure 9-2).
- <u>Open fracture:</u> An open wound exists, and the broken bone end may be protruding through the skin (Figure 9-3).

Recognizing Bone Injuries

It may be difficult to tell if a bone is broken. When in doubt, provide care as if the bone were broken. Any part of the mnemonic DOTS (deformity, open wound, tenderness, swelling) can indicate a sign of a possible fracture:

- *Deformity* might not be obvious. Compare the injured part with the un-injured part on the other side.
- *Open wound* may indicate an underlying fracture.
- *Tenderness* and pain are commonly found only at the injury site. The victim can usually point to the site of the pain or feel pain when it is touched.
- *Swelling* caused by bleeding happens rapidly after a fracture.

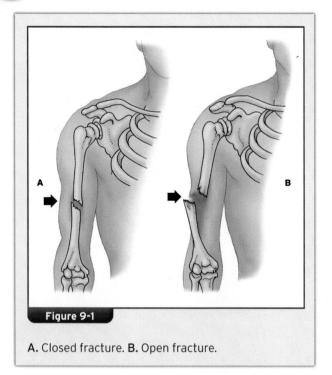

Figure 9-1

A. Closed fracture. **B.** Open fracture.

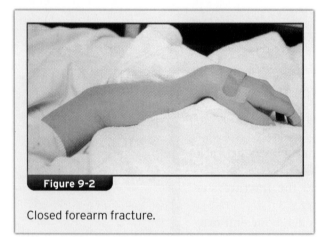

Figure 9-2

Closed forearm fracture.

Additional signs of a fracture include the following:
- The victim is unable to use the injured part normally.
- A grating or grinding sensation can be felt and sometimes even heard when the ends of the broken bone rub together.
- The victim may have heard or felt the bone snap.

Care for Bone Injuries

To care for a bone injury:
1. Expose and examine the injury site.

- Look for deformity, open wounds, bruising, and swelling.
- Feel the injured area for deformity and tenderness when touched.
- Ask the victim about pain and the ability to use the injured part normally.
2. Stabilize the injured part to prevent movement.
   - Follow BSI precautions.
   - If emergency medical services (EMS) will arrive soon, stabilize the injured part with your hands until they arrive.
   - If EMS will be delayed, or if you are taking the victim to medical care, stabilize the injured part with a <u>splint</u> (see Skill Drills 9-1, 9-2, and 9-3).
3. If the injury is an open fracture, do not push on any protruding bone. Cover the wound and exposed bone with a dressing. Place rolls of gauze around the bone, and bandage the injury without applying pressure on the bone.
4. Apply an ice or cold pack if possible to help reduce the swelling and pain.
5. Seek medical care. Call 9-1-1 for any open fractures or large bone fractures (such as the thigh) or when transporting the victim would be difficult or would aggravate the injury.

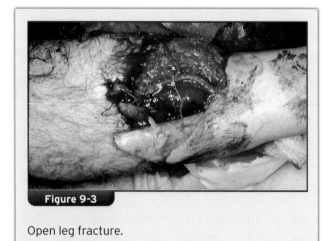

Figure 9-3

Open leg fracture.

▶ Splinting

Splinting an injured area helps:
- Reduce pain
- Prevent further damage to muscles, nerves, and blood vessels

- Prevent a closed fracture from becoming an open fracture
- Reduce bleeding and swelling

Types of Splints

A splint is any device used to stabilize a fracture or a dislocation. Such a device can be improvised (for example, a folded newspaper) or can be a commercially available splint (for example, a SAM splint). Lack of a commercial splint should never prevent you from properly stabilizing an injured extremity.

A rigid splint is an inflexible device such as a padded board, a piece of heavy cardboard, or a SAM splint molded to fit the extremity. It must be long enough so that it can stabilize the area above and below the fracture site **Figure 9-4** .

A soft splint, such as a pillow or rolled blanket, is useful mainly for stabilizing fractures of the ankle **Figure 9-5** .

A self-splint, or anatomic splint, is one in which the injured body part is tied to an uninjured part (for example, an injured finger to the adjacent finger, an injured arm to the chest, or the legs to each other) **Figure 9-6** .

Splinting Guidelines

The following guidelines should be used when splinting.

- Cover any open wounds with a dry dressing before applying a splint.
- Apply a splint only if it does not cause further pain to the victim.

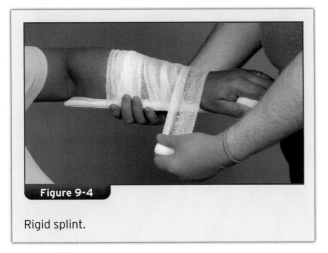

Figure 9-4

Rigid splint.

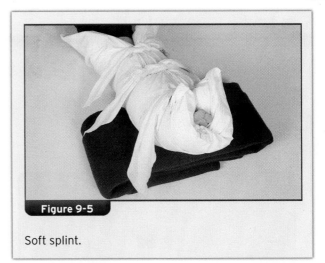

Figure 9-5

Soft splint.

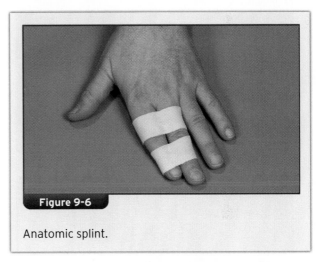

Figure 9-6

Anatomic splint.

- Splint the injured area in the position found.
- The splint should extend beyond the joints above and below an extremity fracture whenever possible.
- Apply splints firmly but not so tightly that blood flow to an extremity is affected.
- Elevate the injured extremity after it is splinted.
- Apply an ice or cold pack.

To splint the lower arm using a self (anatomic) splint, follow the steps in **Skill Drill 9-1** :

1. Use a triangular bandage to create a sling to support the injured arm **(Step ❶)**.
2. Tie the ends of the triangular bandage and secure the sling at the elbow **(Steps ❷a and ❷b)**.
3. Use a triangular bandage folded into a wide binder to secure the sling and the arm to the chest **(Step ❸)**.

skill drill

9-1 Applying a Self (Anatomic) Splint: Lower Arm

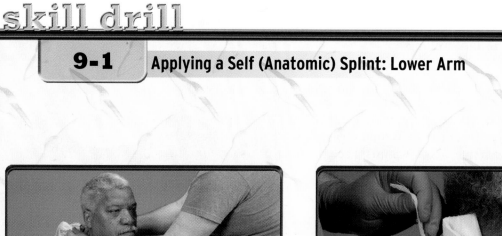

1 Use a triangular bandage to create a sling.

2a Tie the ends of the triangular bandage.

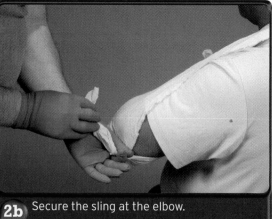

2b Secure the sling at the elbow.

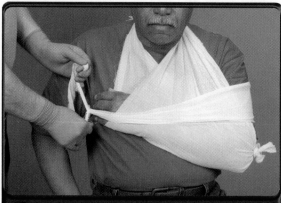

3 Use a triangular bandage folded into a wide binder to secure the sling and the arm to the chest.

To apply a rigid splint to the lower arm, follow the steps in **Skill Drill 9-2** :

1. Place a splint under the injured arm in the position found. A roll of gauze should be placed in the hand to maintain normal position of the hand (Step **1**).
2. Secure the splint with a roll of gauze (Step **2**) or two triangular bandages folded into binders.
3. Use a triangular bandage to create a <u>sling</u> to support the injured arm (Step **3**).
4. Tie the ends of the triangular bandage and secure the sling at the elbow (Step **4**).
5. Use a triangular bandage folded into a wide binder to secure the sling and the splint to the chest. (Step **5**).

To apply a soft splint to the lower arm, follow the steps in **Skill Drill 9-3** :

1. Use a rolled blanket or folded pillow to provide a splint for the injured arm in the position found (Step **1**).
2. Secure the splint with several triangular bandages folded into binders (Step **2**).
3. Use a triangular bandage to create a sling to support the injured arm (Step **3**).
4. Tie the ends of the triangular bandage and secure the sling at the elbow (Steps **4a** and **4b**).
5. Use a triangular bandage folded into a wide binder to secure the sling and the splint to the chest (Step **5**).

Lower leg splints follow the same principles as lower arm splints (see Figure 9-5). If more support is needed, you can bind both legs together.

▶ Joint Injuries

A <u>sprain</u> is a common injury to a joint in which the ligaments and other tissues are damaged by violent stretching or twisting. Attempts to move or use the joint increase the pain. Common locations for sprains include the ankles, wrists, and knees.

A <u>dislocation</u> is a serious and less common joint injury. It occurs when a joint comes apart and stays apart, with the bone ends no longer in contact. The shoulders, elbows, fingers, hips, knees, and ankles are the joints most frequently dislocated.

Recognizing Joint Injuries

The signs of a sprain or dislocation are similar to those of a fracture: pain, swelling, and inability to use the injured joint normally. The main sign of a dislocation is deformity. Its appearance will be different from that of an uninjured joint **Figure 9-7A, B** .

Care for Joint Injuries

To care for a joint injury:

1. If you suspect a dislocation, apply a splint if EMS will be delayed. Provide care as you would for a fracture. Do not try to put the displaced part back into its normal position, because nerve and blood vessel damage could result.
2. If you suspect a sprain, use the RICE procedure (see Skill Drill 9-4).
3. Seek medical care. Call 9-1-1 for any dislocations or injuries for which transporting the victim would be difficult or would aggravate the injury.

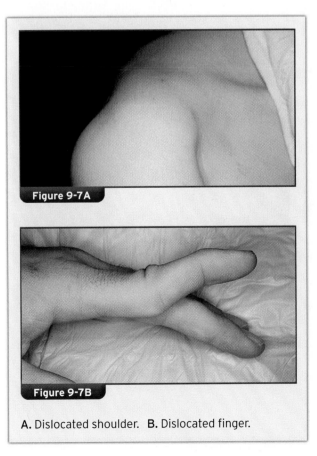

Figure 9-7A

Figure 9-7B

A. Dislocated shoulder. **B.** Dislocated finger.

skill drill

9-2 Applying a Rigid Splint: Lower Arm

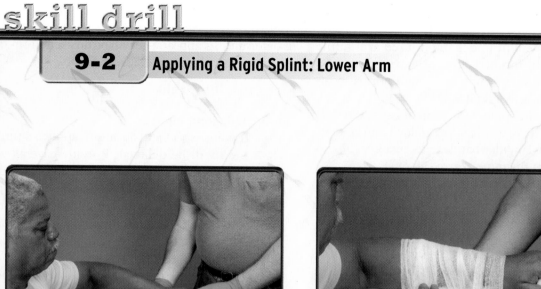

1 Place splint under the injured arm in the position found. Place hand in its normal position.

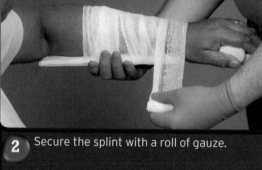

2 Secure the splint with a roll of gauze.

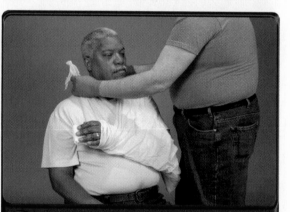

3 Create a sling using a triangular bandage.

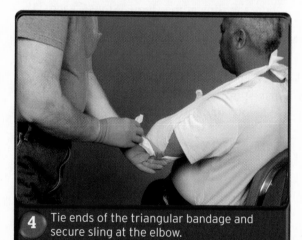

4 Tie ends of the triangular bandage and secure sling at the elbow.

skill drill

9-2   Continued

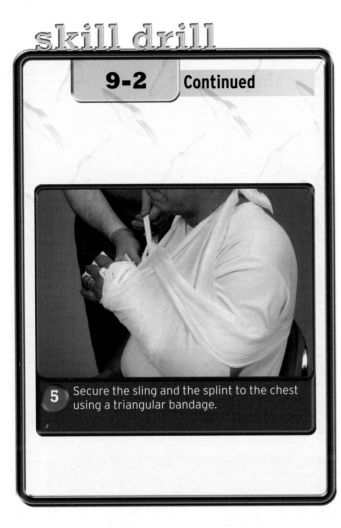

5 Secure the sling and the splint to the chest using a triangular bandage.

▶ RICE Procedure

RICE is the acronym for rest, ice, compression, and elevation. This mnemonic will help you remember the care for a joint injury (for example, a sprain) or a muscle injury (for example, a strain or contusion).

To perform the RICE procedure, follow the steps in **Skill Drill 9-4** :

1. R=Rest. Stop using the injured area.
2. I=Ice. Place an ice pack on the injured area. Use an elastic bandage to hold the ice pack in place for 20 to 30 minutes **(Step ❶)**.
3. C=Compression. Remove the ice and apply a compression bandage and leave in place for 3 to 4 hours **(Step ❷)**.
4. E=Elevation. Raise the injured area higher than the heart, if possible **(Step ❸)**.

R = Rest

Injuries heal faster if the patient rests. Rest means the victim does not use or move the injured part. Using any part of the body increases the blood circulation to that area, which can cause more swelling of an injured part.

I = Ice

An ice or cold pack can be applied to the injured area for 20 to 30 minutes. This should be done every 2 or 3 hours during the first 24 hours.

Cold constricts the blood vessels to and in the injured area, which helps reduce the swelling and inflammation as it dulls the pain and relieves muscle spasms.

To apply cold to an injury, place a thin, wet covering such as a gauze pad or cloth over the injured area and place the ice pack or cold pack on top of the covering. You can use an elastic bandage to hold the ice in place.

C = Compression

Compression reduces internal bleeding and swelling. Following the application of ice or cold, apply an elastic bandage. Start the elastic bandage several inches below the injury and wrap in an upward, overlapping spiral, starting with even and somewhat tight pressure, and then gradually wrap more loosely above the injury. Stretch a new elastic bandage to about one third its maximum length for adequate compression. Leave fingers and toes exposed so possible color change can be easily observed. Pale skin, pain, numbness, and tingling are signs that the bandage is too tight. If any of these symptoms appears, remove the elastic bandage. Leave the elastic bandage off until all the symptoms disappear, then rewrap the area less tightly.

The victim should wear the elastic bandage for the first 18 to 24 hours (except when cold is being applied). At night, the victim should loosen but not remove the elastic bandage.

E = Elevation

Once fluid gets to the hands or feet, it has nowhere else to go and so it causes those body parts to swell. Elevating the injured area, in combination with ice

skill drill

9-3   **Applying a Soft Splint: Lower Arm**

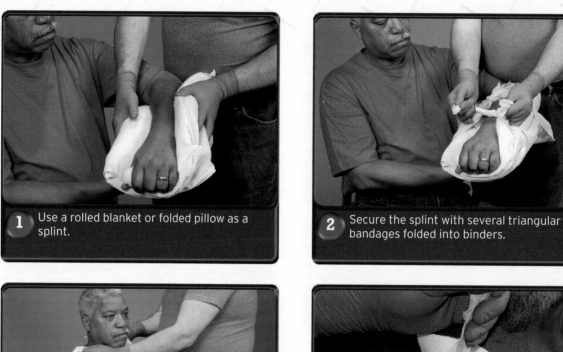

1 Use a rolled blanket or folded pillow as a splint.

2 Secure the splint with several triangular bandages folded into binders.

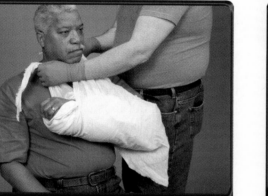

3 Use a triangular bandage to create a sling.

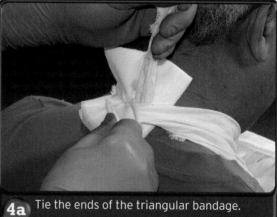

4a Tie the ends of the triangular bandage.

skill drill

9-3 **Applying a Soft Splint: Lower Arm Continued**

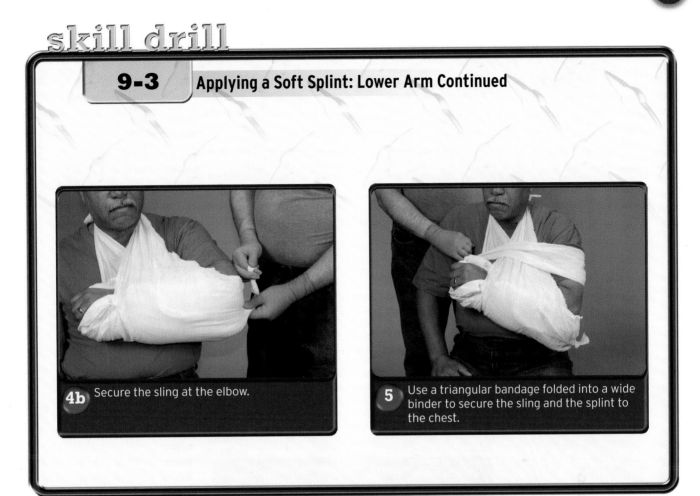

4b Secure the sling at the elbow.

5 Use a triangular bandage folded into a wide binder to secure the sling and the splint to the chest.

Bone, Joint, and Muscle Injuries

Type of Injury Suspected?

Bone Injury

- Expose and examine the injury site.
- Bandage any open wound.
- Splint the injured area.
- Apply an ice or cold pack.
- Seek medical care.

Joint Injury

- Expose and examine the injury site.
- Splint the injured area.
- Apply an ice or cold pack.
- Seek medical care.

Muscle Injury

- Rest.
- Apply an ice or cold pack to muscle strains and contusions.
- Stretch or apply direct pressure to muscle cramps.

skill drill

9-4   RICE Procedure

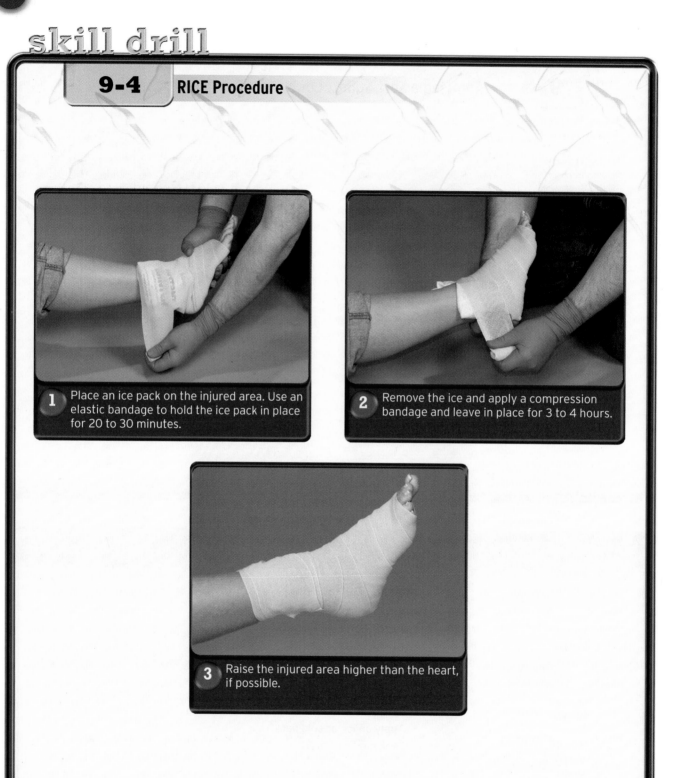

1   Place an ice pack on the injured area. Use an elastic bandage to hold the ice pack in place for 20 to 30 minutes.

2   Remove the ice and apply a compression bandage and leave in place for 3 to 4 hours.

3   Raise the injured area higher than the heart, if possible.

Elevating the injured area, in combination with ice and compression, limits circulation to that area, which in turn helps limit internal bleeding and swelling.

Whenever possible, elevate the injured part above the level of the heart for the first 24 hours after an injury. If a fracture is suspected, do not elevate an extremity until it has been stabilized with a splint.

> **CAUTION**
>
> DO NOT apply an ice or cold pack for more than 30 minutes at a time. Frostbite or nerve damage can result.
>
> DO NOT stop using an ice or cold pack too soon. A common mistake is the early use of heat, which increases circulation to the injured area, resulting in swelling and pain.

▶ Muscle Injuries

A muscle strain, also known as a muscle pull, occurs when a muscle is overstretched and tears. Back muscles are commonly strained when people lift heavy objects.

A muscle contusion, or bruise, results from a blow to the muscle. A muscle cramp occurs when a muscle goes into an uncontrolled spasm.

Recognizing Muscle Injuries

The signs of a muscle strain include the following:
- Sharp pain
- Extreme tenderness when the area is touched
- An indentation or bump that can be felt or seen
- Weakness and loss of function of the injured area
- Stiffness and pain when the victim moves the muscle

The signs of a muscle contusion include the following:
- Pain and tenderness
- Swelling
- Bruise appearing hours after the injury

The signs of a muscle cramp include the following:
- Uncontrolled spasm
- Pain
- Restriction or loss of movement

Care for Muscle Injuries

Care for muscle strains and contusions includes resting the affected muscles and applying an ice or cold pack. To care for a muscle cramp, have the victim stretch the affected muscle or apply pressure directly to it.

> **Meeting OSHA Guidelines**
>
> This chapter covers the following *OSHA Best Practices Guide: Fundamentals of a Workplace First Aid Program (2006)*:
>
> 5. Responding to Non-Life-Threatening Emergencies
>   - Musculoskeletal Injuries
>   - Fractures;
>   - Sprains, strains, contusions and cramps

▶ Bone Injuries

What to Look For

Fractures (broken bones)
- DOTS (deformity, open wound, tenderness, swelling)
- Inability to use injured part normally
- Grating or grinding sensation felt or heard
- Victim heard or felt bone snap

What to Do

1. Expose and examine the injury site.
2. Bandage any open wound.
3. Splint the injured area.
4. Apply ice or cold pack.
5. Seek medical care: Depending on the severity, call 9-1-1 or transport to medical care.

▶ Joint Injuries

What to Look For

Dislocation or sprain
- Deformity
- Pain
- Swelling
- Inability to use injured part normally

What to Do

Dislocation
1. Expose and examine the injury site.
2. Splint the injured area.
3. Apply ice or cold pack.
4. Seek medical care.

Sprain
1. Use RICE procedures.

▶ Muscle Injuries

What to Look For

Strain
- Sharp pain
- Extreme tenderness when area is touched
- Indentation or bump
- Weaknesss and loss of function of injured area
- Stiffness and pain when victim moves the muscle

Contusion
- Pain and tenderness
- Swelling
- Bruise on injured area

Cramp
- Uncontrolled spasm
- Pain
- Restriction or loss of movement

What to Do

1. Use RICE procedures.

1. Use RICE procedures.

1. Stretch and/or apply direct pressure to the affected muscle.

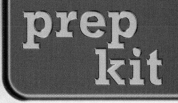

▶ Key Terms

closed fracture A fracture in which there is no laceration in the overlying skin.

contusion A bruise; an injury that causes a hemorrhage in or beneath the skin but does not break the skin.

cramp A painful spasm, usually of a muscle.

dislocation Bone ends at a joint are no longer in contact.

fracture Any break in a bone.

open fracture A fracture exposed to the exterior; an open wound lies over the fracture.

sling Any bandage or material that helps support the weight of an injured upper extremity.

splint A device used to stabilize an injured extremity.

sprain Torn joint ligaments.

strain Stretched or torn muscle.

▶ Assessment in Action

During a softball game, a batter loses his grip while swinging at a pitch. The bat flies through the air and hits a nearby player hard on the arm. Although the skin is not broken, there is tenderness and some swelling.

Directions: Circle Yes if you agree with the statement, and circle No if you disagree.

Yes   No   1. A splint can help stabilize a broken bone against movement.

Yes   No   2. Applying heat reduces bleeding and swelling.

Yes   No   3. A splint should be applied snugly enough to reduce blood flow to the injured area.

Yes   No   4. A fracture should be splinted in the position found.

Yes   No   5. A sling can be applied after splinting an upper extremity fracture.

Answers: 1. Yes; 2. No; 3. No; 4. Yes; 5. Yes

▶ Check Your Knowledge

Directions: Circle Yes if you agree with the statement, and circle No if you disagree.

Yes   No   1. Apply cold on a suspected sprain.

Yes   No   2. The letters RICE stand for rest, ice, compression, and elevation.

Yes   No   3. An elastic bandage, if used correctly, can help control swelling in a joint.

Yes   No   4. A broken leg can be splinted by tying both legs together.

Yes   No   5. A blanket rolled around an ankle is an example of a self (anatomic) splint.

Yes   No   6. A dislocation is cared for much differently than a fracture.

Yes   No   7. Check a suspected fracture by having the victim move the extremity.

Yes   No   8. Treat a muscle cramp by stretching the affected muscle.

Yes   No   9. A pillow can serve as a splint.

Yes   No   10. Do not push on a protruding bone.

Answers: 1. Yes; 2. Yes; 3. Yes; 4. Yes; 5. No; 6. No; 7. No; 8. Yes; 9. Yes; 10. Yes

10

chapter
at a glance

Sudden Illnesses

▶ Heart Attack

A <u>heart attack</u> occurs when the heart muscle tissue dies because its blood supply is reduced or stopped. Usually a clot in a coronary artery (the vessel that carries blood to the heart muscle) blocks the blood supply. The heart stops (known as a cardiac arrest) if a lot of the heart muscle is affected.

Recognizing a Heart Attack

Prompt medical care at the onset of a heart attack is vital to survival and the quality of recovery. This is sometimes easier said than done because many victims deny they are experiencing something as serious as a heart attack. The signs of a heart attack include the following:

- Chest pressure, squeezing, or pain that lasts more than a few minutes or that goes away and comes back. Some victims have no chest pain.
- Pain spreading to the shoulders, neck, jaw, or arms
- Dizziness, sweating, nausea
- Shortness of breath

Most women do not have the classic signs of heart attack seen in men. Instead, they often have severe fatigue, upset stomach, and shortness of breath. Only about one third of women complain of severe chest pain. While cardiovascular disease affects both sexes equally, when women have heart attacks they are more likely than men to die.

Care for a Heart Attack

To care for a heart attack victim:

1. Seek medical care by calling 9-1-1. Medications to dissolve a clot are available but must be given early.
2. Help the victim into the most comfortable resting position **Figure 10-1** .
3. If the victim is alert, able to swallow, and not allergic to aspirin, give one adult aspirin or two to four chewable children's aspirin.
4. If the victim has prescribed medication for heart disease, such as nitroglycerin, help the victim use it.
5. Monitor breathing.

▶ Angina

Angina is chest pain associated with heart disease that occurs when the heart muscle does not get enough blood. Angina is brought on by physical activity, exposure to cold, or emotional stress.

Recognizing Angina

The signs of angina are similar to those of a heart attack, but the pain seldom lasts longer than 10 minutes and almost always is relieved by nitroglycerin (a prescribed medication).

Care for Angina

To care for a victim with angina:

1. Have the victim rest.
2. If a victim has his or her own nitroglycerin, help the victim use it.
3. If the pain continues beyond 10 minutes, suspect a heart attack and call 9-1-1.

▶ Stroke

A stroke, also called a brain attack, occurs when part of the blood flow to the brain is suddenly cut off. This occurs when arteries in the brain rupture or become blocked **Figure 10-2** .

Recognizing Stroke

The signs of a stroke include the following:

- Sudden weakness or numbness of the face, an arm, or a leg on one side of the body
- Blurred or decreased vision, especially on one side of the visual field
- Problems speaking
- Dizziness or loss of balance
- Sudden, severe headache

Care for Stroke

To care for a stroke victim:

1. Call 9-1-1.
2. If the victim is responsive, lay the victim on

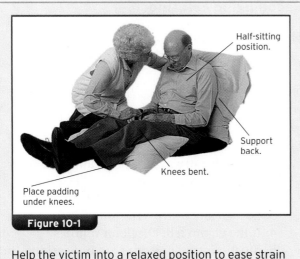

Half-sitting position.

Support back.

Knees bent.

Place padding under knees.

Figure 10-1

Help the victim into a relaxed position to ease strain on the heart.

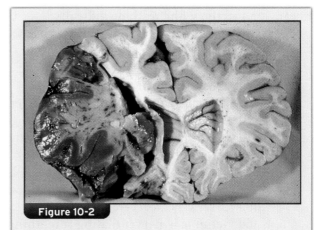

Figure 10-2

Severe brain hemorrhage causing a stroke.

his or her back with the head and shoulders slightly elevated.

3. If the victim is unresponsive, open the airway, check breathing, and provide care accordingly. If the unresponsive victim is breathing, place the victim on his or her side (recovery position) to keep the airway clear.

▶ Breathing Difficulty

Breathing difficulty can result from injuries to the chest or head and from illnesses such as heart attack, anaphylaxis, or asthma. <u>Asthma</u> is a condition in which air passages narrow and mucus builds up, resulting in poor oxygen exchange. It can be triggered by such things as an allergy, cold exposure, and smoke. <u>Hyperventilation</u> is fast breathing, which can be caused by emotional stress, anxiety, and medical conditions.

Recognizing Breathing Difficulty

The signs of breathing difficulty include the following:
- Breathing that is abnormally fast or slow
- Breathing that is abnormally deep (gasping) or shallow
- Noisy breathing, including wheezing (seen with asthma) or gurgling, crowing, or snoring sounds
- Bluish lips
- Need to pause while speaking to catch breath

Care for Breathing Difficulty

To care for a victim with breathing difficulty:
1. Help the victim into the most comfortable position. This is often seated upright.
2. Seek medical care by calling 9-1-1 for sudden, unknown breathing problems.
3. If the victim has a prescribed asthma inhaler, assist the victim in using it **Figure 10-3**. If needed, the victim may use the inhaler again in 5 to 10 minutes.
4. If the victim's condition does not improve following inhaler use, or if the victim's condition worsens, seek medical care by calling 9-1-1.
5. If the victim is hyperventilating (breathing fast) due to anxiety, have him or her inhale through the nose, hold the breath for several seconds, then exhale slowly.

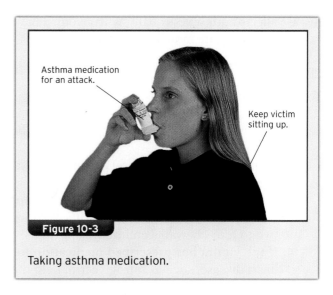

Asthma medication for an attack.

Keep victim sitting up.

Figure 10-3

Taking asthma medication.

CAUTION

DO NOT have a hyperventilating victim breathe into a bag—it does not work and can be dangerous.

▶ Fainting

Fainting can happen suddenly when blood flow to the brain is interrupted. Causes include exhaustion, lack of food, reaction to pain or the sight of blood, hearing bad news, and standing too long without moving.

Recognizing Fainting

The signs of fainting include the following:
- Sudden, brief unresponsiveness
- Pale skin
- Sweating

Care for Fainting

To care for fainting:
1. Open the airway, check breathing, and provide appropriate care.
2. Raise the victim's legs 6 to 12 inches.
3. Loosen any restrictive clothing.
4. If the victim fell, check for injuries.
5. Most fainting episodes are not serious, and the victim recovers quickly. Seek medical care if the victim:

- Has repeated fainting episodes
- Does not quickly become responsive
- Becomes unresponsive while sitting or lying down
- Faints for no apparent reason

▶ Seizures

A seizure results from an abnormal stimulation of the brain's cells. A variety of causes can lead to seizures, including the following:

- Epilepsy
- Heatstroke
- Poisoning
- Electric shock
- Hypoglycemia
- High fever in children
- Brain injury, tumor, or stroke
- Alcohol or other drug withdrawal or abuse

Recognizing Seizure

The signs of a seizure will vary depending on the type of seizure and can include the following:

- Sudden falling
- Unresponsiveness
- Rigid body and arching of the back
- Jerky muscle movement

Care for a Seizure

To care for a victim having a seizure:

1. Prevent injury by moving away any dangerous objects.
2. Loosen any restrictive clothing.
3. Roll the victim onto his or her side (recovery position).
4. Call 9-1-1 if any of the following exists:
   - A seizure occurs for an unknown reason.
   - A seizure lasts more than 5 minutes.
   - The victim is slow to recover, has a second seizure, or has difficulty breathing afterward.
   - The victim is pregnant or has another medical condition.
   - There are any signs of injury or illness.

▶ Diabetic Emergencies

Diabetes results when the body fails to produce sufficient amounts of insulin. Insulin helps regulate blood sugar level. The body cells become starved for sugar. There are two types of diabetes:

- *Type 1:* People with type 1 diabetes require external (not made by the body) insulin to allow sugar to pass from the blood into cells.
- *Type 2:* People with type 2 diabetes are not dependent on external insulin to allow sugar into cells.

The body is continuously balancing sugar and insulin. Too much insulin and not enough sugar leads to low blood sugar (hypoglycemia) and possibly insulin shock. Too much sugar and not enough insulin leads to high blood sugar (hyperglycemia) and possibly diabetic coma **Figure 10-4**.

Recognizing Low Blood Sugar

A very low blood sugar level, called hypoglycemia, can be caused by too much insulin, too little or delayed food intake, exercise, alcohol, or any combination of these factors.

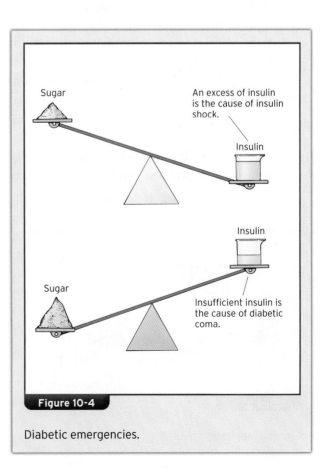

Figure 10-4

Diabetic emergencies.

In a person with diabetes, the signs of low blood sugar include the following:

- Sudden onset
- Staggering, poor coordination
- Anger, bad temper
- Pale skin
- Confusion, disorientation
- Sudden hunger
- Excessive sweating
- Trembling
- Seizures
- Unresponsiveness

Care for Low Blood Sugar

To care for a diabetic with low blood sugar (hypoglycemia) who is responsive and can swallow:

1. Give sugar, such as two large teaspoons or lumps of sugar, half a can of regular soda, 4 ounces of orange juice, three glucose tablets, or one tube of glucose gel Figure 10-5.
2. If there is no improvement after 15 minutes, repeat giving sugar.
3. If there still is no improvement, seek medical care by calling 9-1-1.

If the victim is unresponsive, do not give anything by mouth. Call 9-1-1.

Recognizing High Blood Sugar

Hyperglycemia, which can lead to diabetic coma, is the opposite of hypoglycemia. Hyperglycemia occurs when the body has too much sugar in the blood but is unable to get it to the cells. This condition may be caused by insufficient insulin, overeating, inactivity, illness, stress, or a combination of these factors.

In a person with diabetes, the signs of high blood sugar include the following:

- Gradual onset
- Drowsiness
- Extreme thirst
- Very frequent urination
- Warm and dry skin
- Vomiting
- Fruity, sweet breath odor
- Rapid breathing
- Unresponsiveness

Care for High Blood Sugar

To care for a diabetic with high blood sugar (hyperglycemia):

1. If you are uncertain whether the victim has a high or low blood sugar level, provide care as you would for low blood sugar.
2. If the victim's condition does not improve in 15 minutes, seek medical care by calling 9-1-1.

▶ Emergencies During Pregnancy

Most pregnancies are normal and occur without complications. However, problems sometimes arise, and medical care is required. It is essential that you remain calm, focused, and considerate of the mother during this unforeseen and stressful situation.

Recognizing Emergencies During Pregnancy

The signs of emergencies during pregnancy include the following:

- Vaginal bleeding
- Cramps in the lower abdomen
- Swelling of the face or fingers
- Severe continuous headache
- Dizziness or fainting
- Blurring of vision or seeing spots
- Uncontrollable vomiting

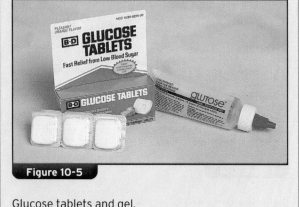

Figure 10-5

Glucose tablets and gel.

Care for Pregnancy Emergencies

If the victim is experiencing vaginal bleeding or abdominal pain or injury:

1. Keep her warm and on her left side.
2. If vaginal bleeding is present, have the victim place a sanitary napkin or any sterile or clean pad over the opening of the vagina.
3. Save any blood-soaked pads and all tissues that are passed. Send this with the woman when she is transported for medical care.
4. Seek medical care.

Sudden Illnesses

Type of Condition Suspected?

Seizure

- Prevent injury.
- Loosen any tight clothing.
- Roll victim onto his or her side.
- Call 9-1-1 if necessary.

Stroke

- Call 9-1-1.
- If responsive, help victim onto his or her back with head and shoulders slightly elevated.
- If unresponsive, move victim onto his or her side.

Fainting

- Check breathing.
- Check for injuries if victim fell.
- Loosen any tight clothing.
- Raise feet 6 to 12 inches.
- Call 9-1-1 if needed.

Diabetic Emergency

If uncertain about high or low blood sugar:

- Give sugar.
- If no improvement in 15 minutes, give more sugar.
- Call 9-1-1 if condition does not improve.

Breathing Difficulty

- Help victim into a comfortable position.
- If asthma attack, help victim with his or her prescribed inhaler medication.
- Call 9-1-1 for unknown cause or asthma not responding to inhaler treatment.
- If breathing fast (hyperventilating) due to anxiety, encourage victim to inhale, hold breath a few seconds, then exhale.

Heart Attack

- Call 9-1-1.
- Help victim into a comfortable position.
- Loosen any tight clothing.
- Give one adult aspirin or two to four children's aspirin.
- Assist victim with his or her prescribed medication.
- Monitor breathing.

Pregnancy Emergencies

If victim is experiencing vaginal bleeding or abdominal pain or injury:

- Keep victim warm.
- For vaginal bleeding, place sanitary napkin or sterile or clean pad over opening of vagina.
- Send blood-soaked pad and tissues with victim to medical care.
- Seek medical care.

▶ Heart Attack

What to Look For

- Chest pressure, squeezing, or pain
- Pain spreading to shoulders, neck, jaw, or arms
- Dizziness, sweating, nausea
- Shortness of breath

What to Do

1. Help victim take his or her prescribed medication.
2. Call 9-1-1.
3. Help victim into a comfortable position.
4. Give one adult or two to four children's aspirin.
5. Monitor breathing.

▶ Angina

What to Look For

- Chest pain similar to a heart attack
- Pain seldom lasts longer than 10 minutes

What to Do

1. Have victim rest.
2. If victim has his or her own nitroglycerin, help the victim use it.
3. If pain continues beyond 10 minutes, suspect a heart attack and call 9-1-1.

▶ Stroke

What to Look For

- Sudden weakness or numbness of the face, an arm, or a leg on one side of the body
- Blurred or decreased vision
- Problems speaking
- Dizziness or loss of balance
- Sudden, severe headache

What to Do

1. Call 9-1-1.
2. If responsive, help victim into a comfortable position with head and shoulders slightly raised.
3. If unresponsive, move onto his or her side.

▶ Breathing Difficulty

What to Look For

- Abnormally fast or slow breathing
- Abnormally deep or shallow breathing
- Noisy breathing
- Bluish lips
- Need to pause while speaking to catch breath

What to Do

Unknown reason
1. Help victim into a comfortable position.
2. Call 9-1-1.

Asthma attack
1. Help victim into a comfortable position.
2. Help victim use inhaler.
3. Call 9-1-1 if victim does not improve.

Hyperventilating
1. Encourage victim to inhale, hold breath a few seconds, then exhale.
2. Call 9-1-1 if condition does not improve.

▶ Fainting

What to Look For

- Sudden, brief unresponsiveness
- Pale skin
- Sweating

What to Do

1. Check breathing.
2. Check for injuries if victim fell.
3. Raise feet 6 to 12 inches.
4. Call 9-1-1 if needed.

▶ Seizures

What to Look For

- Sudden falling
- Unresponsiveness
- Rigid body and arching of back
- Jerky muscle movement

What to Do

1. Prevent injury.
2. Loosen any tight clothing.
3. Roll victim onto his or her side.
4. Call 9-1-1 if needed.

▶ Diabetic Emergencies

What to Look For

Low blood sugar
- Develops very quickly
- Anger, bad temper
- Hunger
- Pale, sweaty skin

High blood sugar
- Develops gradually
- Thirst
- Frequent urination
- Fruity, sweet breath odor
- Warm and dry skin

What to Do

1. If uncertain about high or low sugar level, give sugar.
2. Repeat in 15 minutes if no improvement.
3. Call 9-1-1 if conditions do not improve.

▶ Pregnancy Emergencies

What to Look For

- Vaginal bleeding
- Cramps in lower abdomen
- Swelling of face or fingers
- Severe continuous headache
- Dizziness or fainting
- Blurring of vision or seeing spots
- Uncontrollable vomiting

What to Do

Vaginal bleeding or abdominal pain or injury

1. Keep victim warm.
2. For vaginal bleeding, place sanitary napkin or sterile or clean pad over opening of vagina.
3. Send blood-soaked pad and tissues with victim to medical care.
4. Seek medical care.

prep kit

▶ Key Terms

angina Chest pain caused by a lack of blood to the heart muscle.

asthma An acute spasm of the smaller air passages that causes difficult breathing and wheezing.

diabetes A disease in which the body is unable to use sugar normally because of a deficiency or total lack of insulin.

heart attack Death of a part of the heart muscle.

hyperglycemia Abnormally high blood sugar level.

hyperventilation Abnormally fast breathing.

hypoglycemia Abnormally low blood sugar level.

seizure Sudden violent muscle rigidity and jerky movements (convulsions) resulting from abnormal stimulation of the brain's cells.

stroke A blockage or rupture of arteries in the brain.

▶ Assessment in Action

A 50-year-old coworker is experiencing chest pain and nausea. He says that it started about an hour ago and has not let up. He believes it may just be indigestion. He describes the pain as "something pressing on my chest."

Directions: Circle Yes if you agree with the statement, and circle No if you disagree.

Yes No 1. Have him lie down for 30 minutes to see if the pain subsides.

Yes No 2. Check to see if his pupils are unequal.

Yes No 3. His signs could indicate a heart attack.

Yes No 4. Help the victim take an aspirin, and call EMS.

Yes No 5. Heart attack victims often resist the idea that they need medical care.

Answers: 1. No; 2. No; 3. Yes; 4. Yes; 5. Yes

▶ Check Your Knowledge

Directions: Circle Yes if you agree with the statement, and circle No if you disagree.

Yes No 1. Heart attack victims can experience chest pain.

Yes No 2. You can help the victim of chest pain take his or her nitroglycerin.

Yes No 3. A responsive stroke victim should lie down with his or her head slightly raised.

Yes No 4. Asthma victims may have a prescribed inhaler.

Yes No 5. A victim who is breathing fast (hyperventilation) should be encouraged to breathe slowly by holding inhaled air for several seconds and then exhaling slowly.

Yes No 6. Raise the feet of a person who has fainted 6 to 12 inches.

Yes No 7. Some seizure victims display a rigid arching of the back.

Yes No 8. A person having seizures always requires medical attention.

Yes No 9. If in doubt about the type of diabetic emergency a victim is experiencing, give sugar to a responsive victim who can swallow.

Yes No 10. Nitroglycerin may relieve chest pain associated with angina.

Answers: 1. Yes; 2. Yes; 3. Yes; 4. Yes; 5. Yes; 6. Yes; 7. Yes; 8. No; 9. Yes; 10. Yes

Meeting OSHA Guidelines

This chapter covers the following *OSHA Best Practices Guide: Fundamentals of a Workplace First Aid Program (2006)*:

4. Responding to Life-Threatening Emergencies
   - Assessing and treating a victim who has an unexplained change in level of consciousness or sudden illness.
   - Responding to Medical Emergencies
     - Chest pain;
     - Stroke;
     - Breathing problems;
     - Hypoglycemia in diabetics taking insulin;
     - Seizures;
     - Pregnancy complications;
     - Reduced level of consciousness.

Poisoning

▶ Poisons

A poison (also known as a *toxin*) is any substance that impairs health or causes death by its chemical action when it enters the body or comes in contact with the skin.

▶ Ingested Poisons

Ingested poisoning occurs when the victim swallows a toxic substance. Fortunately, most poisons have little toxic effect or are ingested in such small amounts that severe poisoning rarely occurs. However, the potential for severe or fatal poisoning is always present. About 80% of all poisonings happen by ingesting a toxic substance.

Recognizing Ingested Poisoning

The signs of ingested poisoning include the following:
- Abdominal pain and cramping
- Nausea or vomiting
- Diarrhea
- Burns, odor, or stains around and in the mouth

- Drowsiness or unresponsiveness
- Poison container nearby

Care for Ingested Poisons

To care for victims who have ingested poisons:

1. Determine the following:
   - The age and size of the victim
   - What was swallowed (read container label; save vomit for analysis)
   - How much was swallowed (for example, a dozen tablets)
   - When it was swallowed
2. For a responsive victim, call the poison control center at 1-800-222-1222. Most poisonings can be treated by following the instructions received by telephone from a **poison control center**. Give **activated charcoal** if you have it and if you are advised to do so by the poison control center **Figure 11-1**. The center staff will also advise you whether medical care is needed.
3. For an unresponsive victim, open the victim's airway, check breathing, and treat accordingly. Call 9-1-1. If the victim is breathing, place the victim in the recovery position on his or her left side to delay absorption of the poison and to prevent **aspiration** (inhalation) into the lungs if vomiting begins **Figure 11-2**.

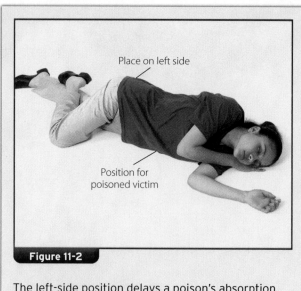

Figure 11-2

The left-side position delays a poison's absorption into the victim's circulatory system.

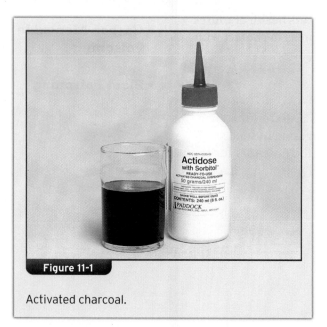

Figure 11-1

Activated charcoal.

FYI

Activated Charcoal

Activated charcoal is a fine, black, odorless powder that is available as a liquid. Activated charcoal prevents the absorption of most poisons and drugs by the stomach and intestines.

Activated charcoal does not absorb all drugs well. Acids and alkalis (for example, bleach and ammonia), potassium, iron, alcohol, methanol, kerosene, and cyanide require different treatment.

A drawback of activated charcoal is its grittiness and its appearance. Trying to improve the taste or consistency by adding chocolate syrup, sherbet, ice cream, or milk only decreases the charcoal's binding capacity.

CAUTION

DO NOT give water or milk to dilute poisons unless instructed to do so by a poison control center.

Ingested Poison

Responsive or Unresponsive Victim?

Responsive Victim

- Call the poison control center for advice (1-800-222-1222).
- Give activated charcoal if instructed to do so.

Unresponsive Victim

- Open airway, check breathing, and treat accordingly.
- If breathing, place the victim on the left side.
- Call 9-1-1.

FYI

Material Safety Data Sheets

For each hazardous chemical in the workplace, an employer is required by law to maintain a copy of the Material Safety Data Sheet (MSDS). An MSDS lists the hazardous ingredients of a product, its physical and chemical characteristics, effects on human health, the chemicals with which it can react adversely, handling precautions, measures that can be used to control exposure and contain a spill, and emergency and first aid procedures.

▶ Alcohol and Other Drug Emergencies

Poisoning caused by an overdose or abuse of medications and other substances, including alcohol, is common. The most commonly abused drug in the United States is alcohol.

Recognizing Alcohol Intoxication

Helping an intoxicated person can be difficult because the person may be belligerent or combative. The victim's condition may be quite serious, even life threatening. Although the following signs indicate alcohol intoxication, some can also mean injury or illness other than alcohol intoxication, such as diabetes:

- The odor of alcohol on a person's breath or clothing
- Unsteadiness, staggering
- Confusion
- Slurred speech
- Nausea and vomiting
- Flushed face

Care for Alcohol Intoxication

To care for alcohol intoxication:

1. If victim is responsive:
   - Monitor breathing.
   - Look for injuries.
   - Place in recovery position (left side).
   - Call poison control center for advice (1-800-222-1222).
   - If victim becomes violent, leave the area and call 9-1-1.
2. If victim is unresponsive, open airway, check breathing, and treat accordingly. Call 9-1-1.

CAUTION

DO NOT let an intoxicated person sleep on his or her back.

DO NOT leave an intoxicated person alone, unless he or she becomes violent.

DO NOT try to handle a hostile intoxicated person by yourself.

Recognizing Drug Overdose

The condition of a person suffering from a drug overdose may be quite serious, even life threatening. The signs of drug overdose include the following:
- Drowsiness, anxiety, agitation, or hyperactivity
- Change in pupil size
- Confusion
- Hallucinations

Care for Drug Overdose

Care for drug overdose is the same as that for alcohol intoxication.

▶ Carbon Monoxide Poisoning

Carbon monoxide (CO) poisoning victims are often unaware of the gas's presence. The gas is invisible, tasteless, odorless, and nonirritating. It is produced by the incomplete burning of organic material such as gasoline, wood, paper, charcoal, coal, and natural gas.

Recognizing Carbon Monoxide Poisoning

It is difficult to determine whether a person is a CO poisoning victim. The signs of CO poisoning include the following:
- Headache
- Ringing in the ears
- Chest pain
- Muscle weakness
- Nausea and vomiting
- Dizziness and visual changes (blurred or double vision)
- Unresponsiveness
- Breathing and heart stopped

The following conditions indicate possible CO poisoning:
- The symptoms come and go.
- The symptoms worsen or improve in certain places or at certain times of the day.
- People around the victim have similar symptoms.
- The symptoms can be confused with the flu.
- Pets seem ill.

Care for Carbon Monoxide Poisoning

To care for victims of carbon monoxide poisoning:

1. Get the victim out of the toxic environment and into fresh air.
2. Call 9-1-1.
3. Monitor breathing.
4. Place an unresponsive breathing victim in the recovery position.

▶ Plant Poisoning

About 50% of people exposed to poison ivy, poison oak, and poison sumac are allergic to the plant and will react to it. More than 60 plants can cause allergic reactions, but poison ivy, poison oak, and poison sumac are by far the most common **Figure 11-3A–C**.

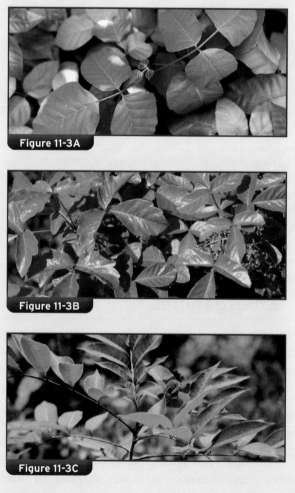

Figure 11-3A

Figure 11-3B

Figure 11-3C

Poisonous plants. **A.** Poison ivy. **B.** Poison oak. **C.** Poison sumac.

Recognizing Plant Poisoning

An allergic reaction may begin as early as 6 hours after contact, but usually it occurs 24 to 72 hours after exposure.

The signs of plant poisoning include the following:

- Rash **Figure 11-4**
- Itching
- Redness
- Blisters
- Swelling

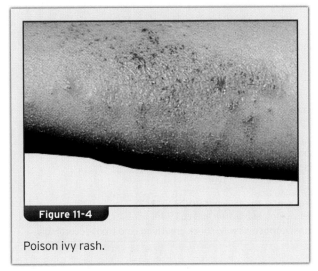

Figure 11-4

Poison ivy rash.

Care for Plant Poisoning

To care for plant poisoning:

1. People who know they have been in contact with a poisonous plant should wash the affected area with soap and cold water as soon as possible to remove oily resin or should apply rubbing (isopropyl) alcohol liberally (not in swab-type dabs).
2. For a mild reaction, have the victim soak in a lukewarm bath sprinkled with 1 to 2 cups of colloidal oatmeal (such as Aveeno) or apply one of the following:
   - Calamine lotion (calamine ointment if the skin becomes dry and cracked)
   - Baking soda paste: 1 teaspoon of water mixed with 3 teaspoons of baking soda
3. For a more severe reaction, care for the skin as you would for a mild reaction and seek medical care. A prescribed oral <u>corticosteroid</u> may be needed.

Meeting OSHA Guidelines

This chapter covers the following OSHA *Best Practices Guide: Fundamentals of a Workplace First Aid Program (2006)*:

4. Responding to Life-Threatening Emergencies
   - Poisoning
     - Ingested poisons: alkali, acid, and systemic poisons. Role of the Poison Control Center (1-800-222-1222);
     - Inhaled poisons: carbon monoxide; hydrogen sulfide; smoke; and other chemical fumes, vapors, and gases. Assessing the toxic potential of the environment and the need for respirators;
     - Knowledge of the chemicals at the worksite and of first aid and treatment for inhalation or ingestion;
     - Effects of alcohol and illicit drugs so that the first aid provider can recognize the physiologic and behavioral effects of these substances.

▶ Poisoning

What to Look For

What to Do

Ingested (swallowed) poisoning
- Abdominal pain and cramping
- Nausea or vomiting
- Diarrhea
- Burns, odor, or stains around and in mouth
- Drowsiness or unresponsiveness
- Poison container nearby

1. Determine the age and size of the victim, what and how much was swallowed, and when it was swallowed.
2. If victim is responsive, call the poison control center at 1-800-222-1222. If advised, give activated charcoal. The center will advise if medical care is needed.
3. If victim is unresponsive, open airway, check breathing, and treat accordingly. If breathing, place on left side in recovery position. Call 9-1-1.

Alcohol intoxication
- Alcohol odor on breath or clothing
- Unsteadiness, staggering
- Confusion
- Slurred speech
- Nausea and vomiting
- Flushed face

1. If the victim is responsive:
   - Monitor breathing.
   - Look for injuries.
   - Place in recovery position.
   - Call poison control center for advice (1-800-222-1222).
   - If victim becomes violent, leave area and call 9-1-1.
2. If victim is unresponsive, open airway, check breathing, and treat accordingly.

Drug overdose
- Drowsiness, agitation, anxiety, hyperactivity
- Change in pupil size
- Confusion
- Hallucinations

1. If the victim is responsive:
   - Monitor breathing.
   - Look for injuries.
   - Place in recovery position.
   - Call poison control center for advice (1-800-222-1222).
   - If victim becomes violent, leave area and call 9-1-1.
2. If victim is unresponsive, open airway, check breathing, and treat accordingly.

Carbon monoxide poisoning
- Headache
- Ringing in ears
- Chest pain
- Muscle weakness
- Nausea and vomiting
- Dizziness and vision difficulties
- Unresponsiveness
- Breathing and heart stopped

1. Move victim to fresh air.
2. Call 9-1-1.
3. Monitor breathing.
4. Place unresponsive breathing victim in recovery position.

Plant (contact) poisoning
- Rash
- Itching
- Redness
- Blisters
- Swelling

1. For known contact, immediately wash with soap and water.
2. For mild reaction, use one or more:
   - 1–2 cups of colloidal oatmeal in bathwater
   - Calamine lotion
   - Baking soda paste
3. For severe reactions, perform step 2 and seek medical care.

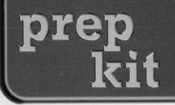

▶ Key Terms

<u>activated charcoal</u> Powdered charcoal that has been treated to increase its powers of absorption. Used to treat patients who have ingested poisons.

<u>aspiration</u> Breathing in foreign matter such as food, drink, or vomitus into the airway or lungs.

<u>carbon monoxide</u> A colorless, odorless, poisonous gas formed by incomplete combustion, such as in fire.

<u>corticosteroid</u> Medication to lessen inflammation and relieve irritation.

<u>ingested poisoning</u> Poisoning caused by swallowing a toxic substance.

<u>Material Safety Data Sheet (MSDS)</u> Lists the hazardous ingredients of products, as well as their characteristics, effects on human health, and treatment for exposure.

<u>poison</u> Any substance that impairs health or causes death by its chemical action when it enters the body or comes in contact with the skin; also known as a toxin.

<u>poison control center</u> Medical facility providing immediate, free, expert advice anytime by calling 1-800-222-1222.

▶ Assessment in Action

You find your 2-year-old son vomiting. You notice that the top of a nearby medicine bottle is off. The label on the bottle reveals that the medicine inside belongs to your mother, who is visiting. You realize that he must have swallowed some of the highly potent medicine.

Directions: Circle Yes if you agree with the statement, and circle No if you disagree.

Yes No 1. Immediately have him drink water or milk.

Yes No 2. Call the poison control center immediately.

Yes No 3. Induce vomiting with ipecac syrup.

Yes No 4. Place him on his left side.

Yes No 5. Give activated charcoal if advised by a poison control center.

Answers: 1. No; 2. Yes; 3. No; 4. Yes; 5. Yes

▶ Check Your Knowledge

Directions: Circle Yes if you agree with the statement, and circle No if you disagree.

Yes No 1. Swallowing a poison can produce nausea.

Yes No 2. Activated charcoal can be used for all victims of ingested poison.

Yes No 3. The best activated charcoal to use is in a capsule form.

Yes No 4. Carbon monoxide has a unique smell.

Yes No 5. Everyone who touches a poison ivy, poison oak, or poison sumac plant will have some type of skin reaction.

Yes No 6. Causing a poisoned victim to vomit is a recommended first aid practice.

Yes No 7. Some cases of poison ivy, poison oak, or poison sumac require medical care.

Yes No 8. Calamine lotion can help relieve itching caused by poison ivy, poison oak, or poison sumac.

Yes No 9. If an intoxicated or drugged person becomes violent, leave the area.

Yes No 10. Move a carbon monoxide victim to fresh air.

Answers: 1. Yes; 2. No; 3. No; 4. No; 5. No; 6. No; 7. Yes; 8. Yes; 9. Yes; 10. Yes

Bites and Stings

▶ Animal and Human Bites

An estimated one of every two Americans will be bitten by an animal or by another person. Dogs account for about 80% of all animal-bite injuries 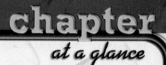.

The human mouth contains a wide range of bacteria, so the chance of infection is greater from a human bite than from bites of other warm-blooded animals.

Rabies

Rabies is caused by a virus found in warm-blooded animals that spreads from one animal to another in the saliva, usually through a bite or lick.

An animal should be considered possibly rabid if:

- The animal attacked without provocation.
- The animal acted strangely or out of character (for example, a usually friendly dog is aggressive or a wild fox seems docile and "friendly").
- The animal was a high-risk species (for example, skunk, raccoon, or bat).

Report animal bites to the police or animal control officers; they should be the ones to capture the animal for observation. If the victim was bitten

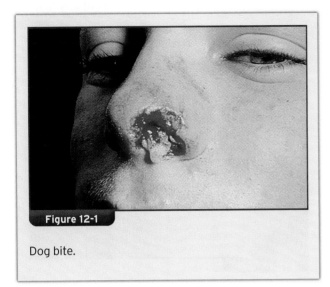

Figure 12-1

Dog bite.

by a healthy domestic dog or cat, the animal should be confined and observed for 10 days for any illness.

If the victim was bitten by a wild animal, the incident should be considered a possible rabies exposure and medical care should be sought immediately.

Care for an Animal Bite

To care for an animal bite:

1. If the wound is not bleeding heavily, wash it with soap and water. Avoid scrubbing, which can bruise the tissues.
2. Flush the wound thoroughly with running water under pressure.
3. Control bleeding and cover the wound with a sterile or clean dressing.
4. Seek medical care for further wound cleaning and closure, and possible tetanus or rabies care.

Care for a Human Bite

To care for a human bite:

1. If the wound is not bleeding heavily, wash it with soap and water under pressure. Avoid scrubbing, which can bruise the tissue.
2. Flush the wound thoroughly with running water under pressure.
3. Control bleeding and cover the wound with a sterile or clean dressing.

4. Seek medical care for further wound cleaning or closure, and possible tetanus care.

CAUTION

DO NOT close a bite wound with tape or butterfly bandages. Closing the wound traps bacteria in the wound, increasing the chance of infection.

▶ Snake Bites

Only four native snake species in the United States are venomous: rattlesnakes (which account for about 65% of all venomous snake bites and nearly all the snake-bite deaths in the United States), copperheads, water moccasins (also known as cottonmouths), and coral snakes. Rattlesnakes **Figure 12-2**, copperheads, and water moccasins are all pit vipers. The coral snake is small and colorful, with a black snout and a series of bright red, yellow, and black bands around its body (every other band is yellow). Venomous snakes from other countries also pose a snake-bite problem.

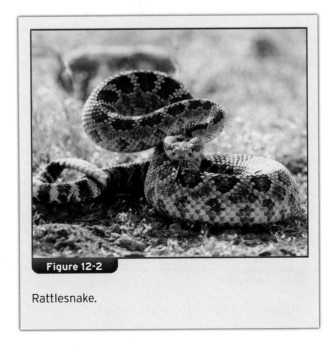

Figure 12-2

Rattlesnake.

Recognizing a Pit Viper Bite

The signs of a pit viper bite include the following:

- Severe, burning pain
- One or two small puncture wounds about one half inch apart **Figure 12-3**
- Swelling
- Discoloration and blood-filled blisters possibly developing hours after the bite **Figure 12-4**
- Nausea, vomiting, sweating, and weakness

FYI

"Dry" Snake Bites
In about 25% of poisonous snake bites, there is no venom injection, only fang and tooth wounds (known as a "dry" bite).

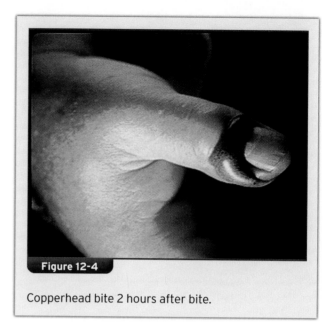

Figure 12-4

Copperhead bite 2 hours after bite.

Care for a Pit Viper Bite

To care for a pit viper bite:

1. Get the victim and bystanders away from the snake.
2. Keep the victim calm and limit movement. If possible, carry the victim or have the victim walk very slowly to help minimize physical exertion.

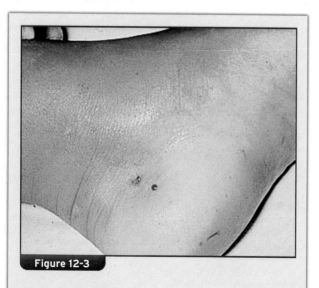

Figure 12-3

Rattlesnake bite (note the two fang marks).

3. Gently wash the bitten area with soap and water.
4. Stabilize a bitten extremity as you would a possible fracture. Keep the extremity below heart level despite the fact that swelling may occur.
5. Seek medical care immediately.

FYI

Antivenin
Identifying the type of pit viper is not very important because the same antivenin is used to counteract all North American pit viper venom.

Recognizing a Coral Snake Bite

The coral snake is America's most venomous snake, but it rarely bites people. The coral snake has short fangs and tends to hang on and "chew" its venom into the victim rather than striking and releasing like a pit viper.

Care for a Coral Snake Bite

To care for a coral snake bite:

1. Get the victim and bystanders away from the snake.

2. Keep the victim calm and limit movement. If possible, carry the victim or have the victim walk very slowly to help minimize physical exertion.
3. Gently wash the bitten area with soap and water.
4. Apply mild pressure (able to slip a finger under it) by wrapping an elastic bandage (for example, an Ace bandage) over the bite site and the entire length of an arm or leg.
5. Seek medical care immediately.

CAUTION

DO NOT cut the victim's skin.
DO NOT attempt to suck out the venom.
DO NOT apply ice or cold to the bitten area.

Recognizing a Nonpoisonous Snake Bite

A nonpoisonous snake leaves horseshoe-shaped tooth marks on the victim's skin. If you are not positive about a snake, assume it was venomous. Some so-called nonpoisonous North American snakes such as hognose and garter snakes have venom that can cause painful local reactions but no systemic (whole-body) symptoms.

Care for a Nonpoisonous Snake Bite

To care for a nonpoisonous snake bite:
1. Get the victim and bystanders away from the snake.
2. Gently wash the bitten area with soap and water.
3. If the wound is minor, apply antibiotic ointment and cover the wound.
4. Seek medical care.

▶ Insect Stings

Severe allergic reactions to insect stings are reported in about 1 in 200 people in the United States yearly **Figure 12-5** . Fortunately, most people will only experience the mild effects of the sting.

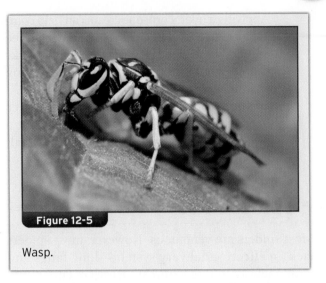

Figure 12-5

Wasp.

Recognizing an Insect Sting

A rule of thumb is that the sooner symptoms develop after a sting, the more serious the reaction will be. Common signs of an insect sting are as follows:
- Pain
- Itching
- Swelling

Signs of a severe allergic reaction (anaphylaxis) include the following:
- Difficulty breathing
- Tightness in the chest
- Itchy, burning skin with a rash or hives
- Swelling of the tongue, mouth, or throat
- Dizziness and nausea

Care for an Insect Sting

To care for an insect sting:
1. If a stinger is embedded (only bees leave their stinger), remove it. Scrape the stinger away with a hard object such as a plastic credit card or driver's license. Do not use tweezers to remove the stinger because they can squeeze more venom into the victim.
2. Wash the area with soap and water.
3. Apply an ice or cold pack over the area to slow absorption of the venom and relieve pain. A baking soda paste may help, except for wasp stings.
4. To further relieve pain and itching, use aspirin (adults only), acetaminophen, or ibuprofen.

Applying a hydrocortisone cream can help combat local swelling and itching. An antihistamine reduces some itching if given early, but it works too slowly to counteract a life-threatening allergic reaction.

5. Observe the victim for at least 30 minutes for signs of a severe allergic reaction. For a person having a severe allergic reaction, call 9-1-1. If the victim has a prescribed auto-injector, help the victim use it.

▶ Spider Bites

Most spiders are venomous. However, most spiders lack an effective delivery system—long fangs and strong jaws—to bite a human. Death occurs rarely and only from bites by brown recluse and black widow spiders. A spider bite is difficult to diagnose, especially when the spider was not seen or recovered, because the bites typically cause little immediate pain.

Recognizing a Black Widow Spider Bite

Black widow spiders have round abdomens that vary from gray to brown to black, depending on the species. The female black widow often has a shiny black abdomen with a red or yellow spot, often in the shape of an hourglass **Figure 12-6**.

Signs of a black widow spider bite can include the following:

- The victim may feel a sharp pinprick when the

spider bites, but some victims are not aware of the bite. Within 15 minutes, a dull, numbing pain develops in the bite area.
- Two small fang marks might be seen as tiny red spots.
- Severe abdominal pain (a bite on an arm can cause severe chest pain, mimicking a heart attack).
- Headache, chills, fever, heavy sweating, dizziness, nausea, and vomiting appear next.

Recognizing a Brown Recluse Spider Bite

Brown recluse spiders are also known in North America as fiddle-back and violin spiders. They have a violin-shaped figure on their backs (several other spider species have a similar configuration on their backs). Color varies from fawn to dark brown, with darker legs **Figure 12-7**.

Brown recluse spiders are found primarily in the southern and midwestern states, with other less toxic but related spiders found throughout the rest of the country. They are absent from the Pacific Northwest, where the aggressive house spider, also known as the hobo spider, is found and causes injuries similar to those of the brown recluse.

Signs of a brown recluse and hobo spider bite include the following:

- A local reaction usually occurs within several hours, with mild to severe pain and itching.
- A blister often develops several days later,

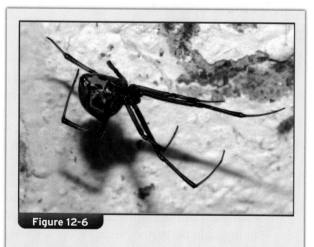

Figure 12-6

Black widow spider. Note red hourglass configuration on abdomen.

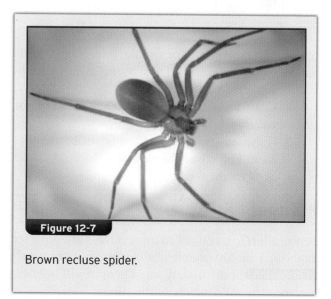

Figure 12-7

Brown recluse spider.

becomes red, and bursts. During the early stages, the affected area often takes on a bull's-eye appearance, with a central white area surrounded by a reddened area, ringed by a whitish or blue border **Figure 12-8** .

- A scab will form that falls off in a few days, leaving a large ulcer. This process of slow tissue destruction can continue for weeks or months. The ulcer sometimes requires skin grafting.
- Other signs can include headache, fever, weakness, nausea, and vomiting.

Recognizing a Tarantula Spider Bite

Tarantulas bite only when provoked or roughly handled. The bite varies from almost painless to a deep throbbing pain that lasts up to 1 hour.

Care for All Spider Bites

To care for any spider bite:

1. If possible, catch the spider to confirm its identity.
2. Wash the bitten area with soap and water or rubbing alcohol.
3. Apply an ice or cold pack over the bite to relieve pain and delay the effects of the venom.
4. Seek medical care. For black widow spider bites, an antivenin exists that can provide relief within a few hours.

▶ Scorpion Stings

Scorpions look like miniature lobsters, with lobster-like pincers and a long upcurved "tail" with a poisonous stinger **Figure 12-9** . Several species of scorpions inhabit the southwestern United States, but only the bark scorpion of Arizona is potentially deadly.

Recognizing a Scorpion Sting

The most frequent sign of a scorpion sting, especially in an adult victim, is local, immediate pain and burning around the sting site. Later, numbness or tingling occurs.

Care for a Scorpion Sting

To care for a scorpion sting:

1. Gently wash the sting site with soap and water or rubbing alcohol.
2. Apply an ice or cold pack over the area.
3. Seek medical care.

▶ Tick Bites

Most tick bites are harmless, although ticks can carry serious diseases **Figure 12-10A, B** . If a tick is carrying a disease, the longer it stays embedded, the greater the chance of disease being transmitted. Because its bite is painless, a tick can remain embedded for days without the victim realizing it.

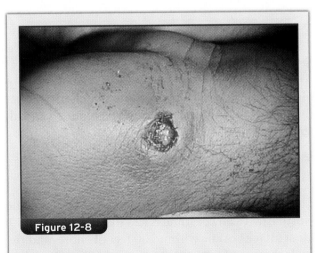

Figure 12-8

Brown recluse spider bite. Note bull's-eye appearance.

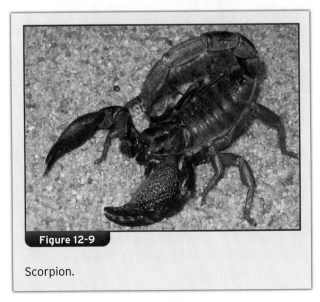

Figure 12-9

Scorpion.

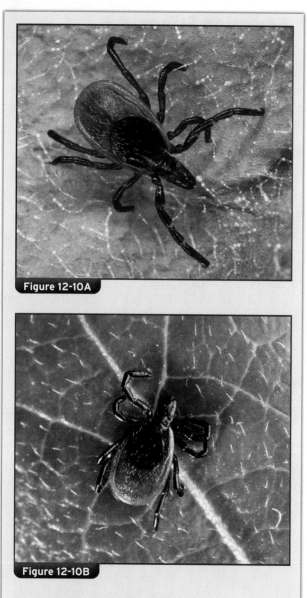

Figure 12-10A

Figure 12-10B

Ticks. **A.** Black-legged tick. **B.** Deer tick.

Care for Tick Bites

1. Remove the tick with tweezers or a specialized tick-removal tool **Figure 12-11**. Grasp the tick as close to the skin as possible and lift the tick with enough force to "tent" the skin surface. Hold it in this position for a minute or until the tick lets go.
2. Wash the area with soap and water. Apply rubbing alcohol.
3. Apply an ice or cold pack to reduce pain.

4. Apply calamine lotion to relieve itching. Keep the area clean.
5. Watch the bitten area for 1 month for a rash, which can be a sign that disease was transmitted by the tick. If a rash appears, seek medical care. Watch for other signs of disease transmitted by ticks, such as fever, muscle or joint aches, and weakness.

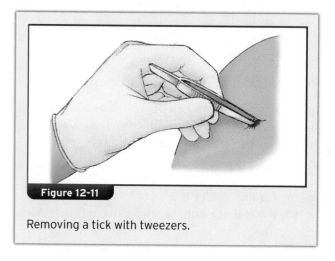

Figure 12-11

Removing a tick with tweezers.

CAUTION

DO NOT use these methods for removing a tick:
- Petroleum jelly
- Fingernail polish
- Gasoline or rubbing alcohol
- Blown-out hot match

▶ Marine Animal Injuries

Most marine animals bite or sting in defense, rather than attacking. Injuries can include wounds and allergic reactions.

Marine Animals that Bite, Rip, or Puncture

The chance of being attacked by a shark along the North American coastline is less than 1 in 5,000,000. Most attacks occur within 100 feet of shore, and the leg is the most frequently bitten body part. Shark bite wounds are similar to injuries caused by boat propellers and chain saws.

Barracudas have an undeserved reputation as attackers of humans. The risk of a barracuda bite is exceedingly small.

Moray eels are known to bite divers who handle or tease them, usually in competition for food or in pursuit of lobsters.

Care for Bites, Rips, or Punctures from Marine Animals

To care for a bite, rip, or puncture caused by a marine animal:

1. Control bleeding.
2. Care for shock.
3. Call 9-1-1.

Marine Animals that Sting

Stings from marine animals lead the list of adverse marine animal encounters. It is important to identify the offending animal, because in many cases care is quite specific.

Each year, jellyfish and Portuguese man-of-wars sting more than 1 million people. Reactions to being stung vary from mild dermatitis to severe reactions. Most victims recover without medical care.

Jellyfish and Portuguese man-of-war stings usually result in welts with redness, burning pain, and muscle cramping. This reaction is due to venom injected by special cells called nematocysts.

Care for Stings from Marine Animals

To care for stings from marine animals:

1. Scrape off any tentacles remaining on the skin. For large tentacles, use tweezers or pliers.
2. Apply vinegar to neutralize nematocysts.

Marine Animals that Puncture by Spines

Stingrays, commonly found in tropical and subtropical waters, are peaceful, reclusive bottom feeders that generally lie buried in the sand or mud. Most wounds inflicted by stingrays are produced on the ankle or foot when the victim steps on a ray. The sting is usually more like a laceration because the large tail barb can do significant damage. The venom causes intense burning pain at the site.

CAUTION

DO NOT try to rub the tentacles off of the victim's skin—rubbing activates the stinging cells.
DO NOT use fresh water for rinsing or ice packs, because it will cause the nematocysts to fire.
DO NOT touch the tentacles with your bare hands.

Care for Punctures from Marine Animal Spines

To care for punctures from marine animal spines:

1. Relieve pain by immersing the injured body part in hot water for 30 to 90 minutes (hot water helps to neutralize the venom). Make sure the water is not hot enough to cause a burn.
2. Wash the wound with soap and water.
3. Flush the area with water under pressure to wash out as much of the toxin and foreign material as possible.
4. Care for the wound.

Meeting OSHA Guidelines

This chapter covers the following *OSHA Best Practices Guide: Fundamentals of a Workplace First Aid Program (2006)*:

5. Responding to Non-Life-Threatening Emergencies
   • Bites and Stings
     • Human and animal bites
     • Bites and stings from insects; instruction in first aid treatment of anaphylactic shock.

▶ Bites and Stings

What to Look For

What to Do

Animal and human bites
- Torn tissue
- Bleeding

1. Wash wound with soap and water.
2. Flush wound thoroughly with water under pressure.
3. Control bleeding.
4. Seek medical care.

Poisonous snake bites
- Severe, burning pain
- Small puncture wounds
- Swelling
- Nausea, vomiting, sweating, weakness
- Discoloration and blood-filled blisters developing hours after the bite

1. Get away from the snake.
2. Limit victim's movement and keep bitten extremity below heart level.
3. Call 9-1-1.
4. Gently wash area with soap and water.
5. For a coral snake bite, apply mild pressure by wrapping the entire affected arm or leg with an elastic bandage.

Insect stings
- Pain
- Itching
- Swelling
- Severe allergic reaction, including breathing problems

1. Scrape away any stinger.
2. Wash with soap and water.
3. Apply an ice or cold pack.
4. Give pain medication, hydrocortisone cream, and an antihistamine.
5. Observe for at least 30 minutes for signs of severe allergic reaction. Call 9-1-1 if a severe allergic reaction occurs. If victim has an epinephrine auto-injector, help victim use it.

Spider bites
- Black widow
  - May feel sharp pain
  - Two small fang marks
  - Severe abdominal pain
  - Headache, chills, fever, sweating, dizziness, nausea
- Brown recluse and hobo
  - Blister developing several days later
  - Ulcer in skin
  - Headache, fever, weakness, nausea

1. Catch spider for identification.
2. Wash bitten area with soap and water.
3. Apply an ice or cold pack.
4. Seek medical care.

Scorpion stings
- Pain and burning at sting site
- Later, numbness or tingling

1. Wash sting site with soap and water.
2. Apply an ice or cold pack.
3. Seek medical care.

Tick bites
- Tick still attached
- Rash (especially one shaped like a bull's-eye)
- Fever, joint aches, weakness

1. Remove tick.
2. Wash bitten area with soap and water.
3. Apply rubbing alcohol.
4. Apply an ice or cold pack.
5. Watch bitten area for 1 month for rash. Seek medical care if rash or other signs such as fever or muscle joint aches appear.

▶ Marine Animal Injuries

What to Look For	What to Do
Bites, rips, or punctures from marine animals (for example, sharks, barracudas, moray eels)	1. Control bleeding. 2. Care for shock. 3. Call 9-1-1.
Stings from marine animals (for example, jellyfish, Portuguese man-of-war)	1. Scrape off tentacles. 2. Apply vinegar.
Punctures from marine animal spines (for example, stingray)	1. Immerse injured part in hot water for 30 to 90 minutes. 2. Wash with soap and water. 3. Flush with water under pressure. 4. Care for wound.

prep kit

▶ Key Terms

<u>antivenin</u> An antiserum containing antibodies against reptile or insect venom.

<u>rabies</u> An acute viral infection of the central nervous system transmitted by the bite of an infected animal.

▶ Assessment in Action

A child has been attacked by a large dog at a local park. The dog has run off into the woods. At least one bystander recognized the dog and believes she knows the owner. You find several dog bite marks on the child's legs and arms.

Directions: Circle Yes if you agree with the statement and circle No if you disagree.

Yes	No	1. Seek medical care for the child.
Yes	No	2. You should call animal control or the police.
Yes	No	3. The dog should be observed for possible rabies.
Yes	No	4. You should control bleeding and care for shock.
Yes	No	5. Dogs account for most of the animal bite injuries.

Answers: 1. Yes; 2. Yes; 3. Yes; 4. Yes; 5. Yes

▶ Check Your Knowledge

Directions: Circle Yes if you agree with the statement and circle No if you disagree.

Yes	No	1. Severe abdominal pain is a sign of a black widow spider bite.
Yes	No	2. Apply an ice or cold pack over a snake bite.
Yes	No	3. Use the "cut and suck" method for a snake bite.
Yes	No	4. Remove a bee's stinger by using tweezers to pull it out.
Yes	No	5. Apply an ice or cold pack over an insect sting or a suspected spider bite.
Yes	No	6. A baking soda paste can help reduce the itching and swelling from an insect sting.
Yes	No	7. A victim's prescribed auto-injector may have to be used if the victim has a life-threatening reaction to an insect sting.
Yes	No	8. Care for stings from marine animals (for example, jellyfish) by pouring hydrogen peroxide on the affected area.
Yes	No	9. Covering an embedded tick with petroleum jelly causes the tick to back out because of the lack of oxygen.
Yes	No	10. Ticks can transmit disease.

Answers: 1. Yes; 2. No; 3. No; 4. No; 5. Yes; 6. Yes; 7. Yes; 8. No; 9. No; 10. Yes

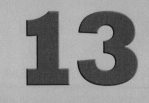

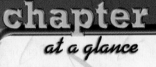

Heat- and Cold-Related Emergencies

▶ Heat-Related Emergencies

Prolonged exposure to high temperatures or physical activity in a hot environment can cause these heat-related illnesses: heat cramps, heat exhaustion, and heatstroke.

Recognizing Heat Cramps

Heat cramps are painful muscle spasms that occur suddenly. They usually involve the muscles in the back of the leg (calf and hamstring muscles) but may also involve the abdomen.

The signs of heat cramps include the following:
- Painful muscle spasms during or after physical activity

Care for Heat Cramps

To care for heat cramps:
1. Have the victim stop activity and rest in a cool area.
2. Stretch the cramped muscle.
3. Remove any excess or tight clothing.
4. If the victim is responsive and not nauseated, provide water or a commercial sports drink (such as Gatorade or Powerade).

Recognizing Heat Exhaustion

<u>Heat exhaustion</u> is caused by the loss of water and salt through heavy sweating. Heat exhaustion affects those who do not drink enough fluid while working or exercising in hot environments and those not acclimated to hot, humid conditions.

The signs of heat exhaustion can include the following:
- Heavy sweating
- Severe thirst
- Weakness
- Headache
- Nausea and vomiting

Care for Heat Exhaustion

To care for heat exhaustion:
1. Have the victim stop activity and rest in a cool area.
2. Remove any excess or tight clothing.
3. If the victim is responsive and not nauseated, provide water or a commercial sports drink.
4. Have the victim lie down and raise legs 6 to 12 inches.
5. Cool the victim by applying cool, wet towels to the victim's head and body.
6. Seek medical care if the condition does not improve within 30 minutes.

Recognizing Heatstroke

<u>Heatstroke</u> is a life-threatening condition in which the body becomes dangerously overheated. Heatstroke can occur quickly (for example, to a long-distance runner during a very hot day) or it can take days to develop (for example, to an elderly person without air conditioning during a heat wave).

The signs of heatstroke can include the following:
- Extremely hot skin
- Dry skin (may be wet at first)
- Confusion
- Seizures
- Unresponsiveness

Care for Heatstroke

To care for heatstroke:
1. Have the victim stop activity and rest in a cool area.

2. Call 9-1-1.
3. If unresponsive, open the airway, check breathing, and provide appropriate care.
4. Rapidly cool the victim by whatever means possible: cool, wet towels or sheets to the head and body accompanied by fanning, and/or cold packs against the armpits, sides of neck, and groin **Figure 13-1** .

► Cold-Related Emergencies

When exposed to very cold environments, the body may become overwhelmed. Cold exposure may cause injury to parts of the body (frostbite) or to the body as a whole (hypothermia).

Recognizing Frostbite

<u>Frostbite</u> happens only when temperatures drop below freezing. It affects mainly the feet, hands, ears, and nose **Figure 13-2A, B** . When skin tissue dies (gangrene) from frostbite, an affected part may have to be amputated.

The signs of frostbite include the following:
- White, waxy-looking skin
- Skin feels cold and numb (pain at first, followed by numbness)
- Blisters, which may appear after rewarming **Figure 13-3**

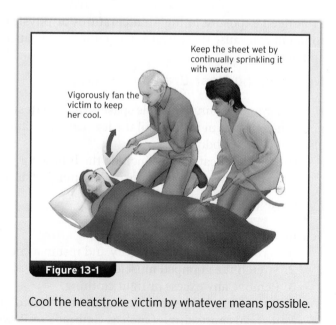

Keep the sheet wet by continually sprinkling it with water.

Vigorously fan the victim to keep her cool.

Figure 13-1

Cool the heatstroke victim by whatever means possible.

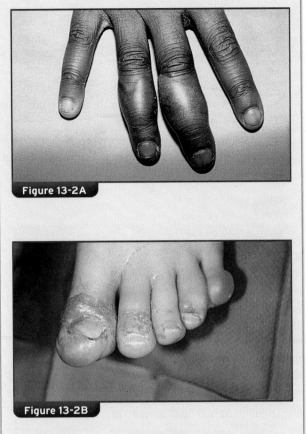

Figure 13-2A

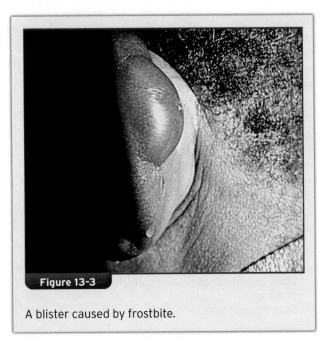

Figure 13-2B

A. Frostbitten fingers. **B.** Frostbitten toes.

Figure 13-3

A blister caused by frostbite.

Care for Frostbite

To care for frostbite:

1. Move the victim to a warm place.
2. Remove tight clothing or jewelry from the injured part.
3. Place dry dressings between the toes and the fingers Figure 13-4 .
4. Seek medical care.

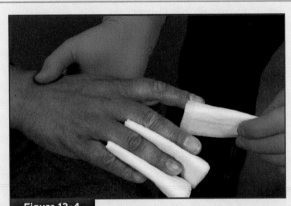

Figure 13-4

Place dry dressings between frostbitten fingers.

CAUTION

DO NOT rub or massage the frostbitten area.

FYI

Caring for Frostbite in a Remote Location

If the victim is in a remote location (more than 1 hour from medical care) and you have warm water, use the following rapid rewarming method:

1. Place the frostbitten part in warm (100°F) water for 20 to 40 minutes or until the tissue becomes soft. For ear or facial injuries, apply warm, moist cloths and change them frequently.
2. After thawing:
   - Place dry dressings between fingers or toes.
   - Slightly elevate the affected part to reduce pain and swelling.
   - Provide aspirin (adults only), ibuprofen, or acetaminophen for pain and swelling.

Recognizing Hypothermia

Hypothermia develops when the body's temperature drops more than 2°F (to about 95°F).

Hypothermia can develop either quickly (for example, cold water immersion) or gradually during prolonged exposure to a cold environment. The temperature does not have to be below freezing for hypothermia to occur.

The signs of hypothermia include the following:
- Uncontrollable shivering
- Confusion, sluggishness
- Cold skin even under clothing

Care for Hypothermia

To care for hypothermia:
1. Get the victim out of the cold.

CAUTION

If the victim is shivering, DO NOT stop it by adding heat (for example, with hot water bottles or heat packs). Shivering generates heat and will rewarm victims with mild hypothermia. Adding heat to the body should only be done at a hospital or a remote location.

2. Prevent heat loss by:
   - Replacing wet clothing with dry clothing
   - Covering the victim's head
   - Placing insulation (such as blankets, towels, coats) beneath and over the victim
3. Have the victim lie down.
4. If the victim is alert and able to swallow, give him or her warm, sugary beverages.
5. Seek medical care for severe hypothermia (rigid muscles, cold skin on abdomen, confusion, lethargy).

FYI

An Ounce of Prevention
Prepare appropriately for any environment.
For a hot environment:
- Wear lightweight, loose-fitting clothes and a hat with a wide brim.
- Drink adequate water or commercial sports drinks.
- Take breaks in cooler areas.

For a cold environment:
- Layer clothing, with moisture-wicking clothing near the skin and outer layers that are wind-proof and waterproof but breathable material.
- Keep head and neck covered to minimize heat loss.
- Drink warm drinks and eat properly.

Heat- and Cold-Related Emergencies

Type of Emergency?

Heat-Related Emergency

- Stop activity and rest.
- Move the victim to a cool area.
- If responsive:
  - Provide water or sports drink if not nauseated.
  - Cool the victim.
  - Call 9-1-1 if the condition does not improve after 30 minutes or worsens.
- If unresponsive:
  - Call 9-1-1.
  - Open the airway, check breathing, and provide appropriate care.
  - Cool the victim rapidly if you suspect heatstroke.

Cold-Related Emergency

- If hypothermia is suspected:
  - Move the victim to a warm area.
  - Replace any wet clothing with dry clothing.
  - Wrap the victim in a blanket.
  - Seek medical care for severe hypothermia.
- If frostbite is suspected:
  - Move the victim to a warm area.
  - Remove tight clothing or jewelry from affected part(s).
  - Place dry dressings between affected fingers or toes.
  - Seek medical care.

▶ Heat-Related Emergencies

What to Look For

What to Do

Heat cramps
- Painful muscle spasm during or after physical activity
- Usually lower leg affected

1. Move victim to cool place.
2. Stretch the cramped muscle.
3. Remove excess or tight clothing.
4. If the victim is responsive, give water or sports drink.

Heat exhaustion
- Heavy sweating
- Severe thirst
- Weakness
- Headache
- Nausea and vomiting

1. Move victim to cool place.
2. Have victim lie down and raise legs 6 to 12 inches.
3. Apply cool, wet towels to head and body.
4. If victim is responsive, give water or sports drink.
5. Seek medical care if no improvement within 30 minutes.

Heatstroke
- Extremely hot skin
- Dry skin (may be wet at first)
- Confusion
- Seizures
- Unresponsiveness

1. Move victim to cool place.
2. Call 9-1-1.
3. If unresponsive, open airway, check breathing, and provide appropriate care.
4. Rapidly cool victim by whatever means possible (cool, wet sheets; ice or cold packs against armpits, side of neck, and groin).

▶ Cold-Related Emergencies

What to Look For

What to Do

Frostbite
- White, waxy-looking skin
- Skin feels cold and numb (pain at first, followed by numbness)
- Blisters, which may appear after rewarming

1. Move victim to warm place.
2. Remove tight clothing or jewelry from injured part(s).
3. Place dry dressings between toes and/or fingers.
4. Seek medical care.

Hypothermia
- Mild
  - Uncontrollable shivering
  - Confusion, sluggishness
  - Cold skin even under clothing
- Severe
  - No shivering
  - Muscles stiff and rigid
  - Skin ice cold
  - Appears to be dead

All victims:
1. Move victim to warm place.
2. Prevent heat loss by
   - Replacing wet clothing with dry clothing
   - Covering victim's head

Mild
1. Give warm, sugary beverages.
2. Do not add anything warm to the skin—let the shivering rewarm the body.

Severe
1. Do not rewarm unless in a very remote location.
2. Call 9-1-1.

prep kit

▶ Key Terms

frostbite Tissue damage caused by extreme cold.

heat cramps Painful muscle spasms, often in the legs.

heat exhaustion Condition caused by the loss of the body's water and salt through excessive sweating.

heatstroke Condition in which the body's heat-regulating ability becomes overwhelmed and ceases to function properly, resulting in an inability to sweat and a dangerously high body temperature.

hypothermia A dangerous condition caused by severe exposure to cold in which the core body temperature drops below 95°F.

▶ Assessment in Action

It is a cold winter weekend, and you feel the need to check on an elderly relative who lives alone. The front door is unlocked, and upon entering her home you notice that it is not much warmer inside the house than outside. You find her wrapped in a blanket lying on the couch. You speak to her, but she only mumbles. She is shivering severely.

Directions: Circle Yes if you agree with the statement, and circle No if you disagree.

Yes   No   1. Add insulation (blankets) around and under her.

Yes   No   2. Shivering can rewarm a victim suffering mild hypothermia.

Yes   No   3. Apply a heating pad immediately.

Yes   No   4. It is too warm in the house for hypothermia to develop.

Yes   No   5. Call 9-1-1 if the condition does not improve in minutes.

Answers: **1.** Yes; **2.** Yes; **3.** No; **4.** No; **5.** Yes

▶ Check Your Knowledge

Directions: Circle Yes if you agree with the statement, and circle No if you disagree.

Yes   No   1. For heat cramps in the legs, stretch the cramped muscle.

Yes   No   2. Commercial sport drinks can be given to victims of heat-related emergencies.

Yes   No   3. Move victims of heat-related illness to a cool place.

Yes   No   4. Victims of heatstroke need immediate medical care—it is a life-threatening condition.

Yes   No   5. Cool heatstroke victims rapidly, including the use of ice packs applied to the neck, armpits, and groin.

Yes   No   6. Rub a frostbitten part to rewarm it.

Yes   No   7. Rewarm a hypothermic victim quickly in a hot shower or with chemical heat packs.

Yes   No   8. Replace any wet clothing with dry clothing for a hypothermic victim.

Yes   No   9. Seek medical care for a severe hypothermic victim.

Yes   No   10. Hypothermia requires below freezing temperatures for it to occur.

Answers: **1.** Yes; **2.** Yes; **3.** Yes; **4.** Yes; **5.** Yes; **6.** No; **7.** No; **8.** Yes; **9.** Yes; **10.** No

Meeting ○SHA Guidelines

This chapter covers the following *OSHA Best Practices Guide: Fundamentals of a Workplace First Aid Program (2006)*:

5. Responding to Non-Life-Threatening Emergencies
   • Temperature Extremes
     • Exposure to cold, including frostbite and hypothermia;
     • Exposure to heat, including heat cramps, heat exhaustion and heat stroke.

Rescuing and Moving Victims

▶ Water Rescue

"Reach-throw-row-go" identifies the sequence for attempting a water rescue:

- If the victim is within reach, extend your arm or an object such as a pole or long stick.
- If the victim is slightly farther away, throw anything that floats (such as a life jacket or throw line).
- If the victim is out of throwing range and there is a boat (such as a canoe, kayak, or rowboat), row to the victim. You could also paddle to the victim using a surfboard or boogie board, or use a motorized water craft if available. Wear a personal flotation device (PFD) for your own safety.
- If none of these procedures is possible and you are trained in water lifesaving procedures, you might swim to the victim.

CAUTION

DO NOT swim to and grasp a drowning person unless you are trained to make the rescue.

▶ Ice Rescue

If a person has fallen through the ice near the shore:

- Extend a pole or throw a line with a floatable object attached to it. When the person has hold of the object, pull him or her toward the shore or the edge of the ice.

CAUTION

DO NOT go near broken ice without support.

▶ Electrical Emergency Rescue

- Most indoor electrocutions are caused by faulty electrical equipment or careless use of electrical appliances. Before you touch the victim, turn off the electricity at the circuit breaker, fuse box, or outside switch box.
- If the electrocution involves high-voltage power lines, the power must be turned off before anyone approaches the victim. Wait for trained personnel with the proper equipment to cut the wires or disconnect them.
- If a power line has fallen over a car, tell the driver and passengers to stay still in the car. A victim should attempt to jump out of the car only if an explosion or fire threatens his or her life. The victim must not make contact with the car or the wire.

CAUTION

DO NOT touch an appliance or the victim until the current is off.

DO NOT try to move downed wires.

DO NOT use any object, even dry wood (for example, broomstick, tools, chair, stool), to separate the victim from the electrical source.

▶ Hazardous Materials Incidents

Almost any highway crash scene involves the potential danger of hazardous chemicals. Clues that indi-

cate the presence of hazardous materials include signs on vehicles (for example, Explosive, Flammable, or Corrosive), spilled liquids or solids, strong, unusual odors, and clouds of vapor **Figure 14-1**. Stay well away and upwind from the area. Only people who are specially trained in handling hazardous materials and who have the proper equipment should be in the area.

▶ Motor Vehicle Crashes

1. Stop and park your vehicle in a safe area. Call 9-1-1.
2. Turn on your vehicle's emergency hazard flashers. Raise the hood of your vehicle to draw more attention to the scene.
3. Make sure everyone at the scene is safe.
4. Ask the driver(s) to turn off the ignition of the involved car(s), or turn it off yourself.
5. Place flares or reflectors 250 to 500 feet behind the crash scene to warn oncoming drivers of the crash. Do not ignite flares around leaking gasoline or diesel fuel.

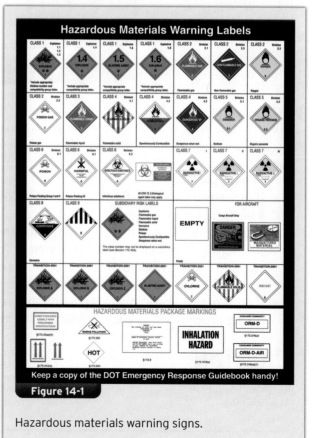

Figure 14-1

Hazardous materials warning signs.

6. If you suspect a victim has a spinal injury, use your hands to stabilize the person's head and neck.
7. Check and care for any life-threatening injuries first, and then handle lesser injuries.

> **CAUTION**
>
> DO NOT rush to get victims out of a car that has been in a crash. Most vehicle crashes do not involve fire, and most vehicles stay in an upright position.
>
> DO NOT move or allow victims to move unless there is an immediate danger, such as fire or oncoming traffic.
>
> DO NOT transport victims in your car or any other bystander's vehicle.

▶ Fires

1. Get all people out of the area quickly.
2. Call 9-1-1.
3. If the fire is small and your own escape route is clear, fight the fire yourself with a fire extinguisher.
4. To use a fire extinguisher, aim directly at the base of the flames of whatever is burning and sweep across it. Extinguishers expel their contents quickly: in 8 to 25 seconds for most home models containing dry chemicals.

▶ Confined Spaces

A confined space is an area not intended for human occupancy that may have or develop a dangerous atmosphere. Below-ground confined spaces include manholes, utility vaults, storage tanks, old mines, and wells. Ground-level confined spaces include industrial tanks and farm storage silos. Above-ground confined spaces include water towers and storage tanks.

An emergency in a confined space demands immediate action. If someone enters a confined space and signals for help or becomes unresponsive, follow these steps:

1. Call 9-1-1.
2. Check motionless victims first. Do not enter the confined space unless you have the proper train-

ing and equipment, such as a self-contained air supply, safety harness, and lifeline.
3. Once the victim is removed, provide care.

▶ Triage: What to Do With Multiple Victims

You may encounter emergency situations in which there is more than one victim. If the scene is safe, decide who must be cared for first. This process of prioritizing or classifying multiple victims is called <u>triage</u>.

To find those needing immediate care for life-threatening conditions, ask all victims who can get up and walk to move to a specific area. Victims who can get up and walk rarely have life-threatening injuries. These victims are known as the "walking wounded." Do not force a victim to move if he or she complains of pain.

Check motionless victims first by opening the airway and checking breathing. You must move rapidly (spend less than 60 seconds with each victim) from one victim to the next until all have been checked. Classify victims according to the following care and transportation priorities:

1. *Immediate care:* Victim needs immediate care and transport to medical care as soon as possible.
   - Breathing difficulties
   - Severe bleeding
   - Severe burns
   - Signs of shock
   - Unresponsiveness
2. *Delayed care:* Care and transportation can be delayed up to 1 hour.
   - Burns without airway problems
   - Major or multiple bone or joint injuries
   - Back injuries with or without suspected spinal cord damage
3. *Walking wounded:* Care and transportation can be delayed up to 3 hours.
   - Minor fractures
   - Minor wounds
4. *Dead:* Victim is obviously dead or unlikely to survive because of the type or extent of injuries.

Do not become involved in providing care for each victim at this point, but ask willing bystanders to assist with such things as bleeding control. Only after victims with immediate life-threatening conditions receive care should people with less serious conditions be given care. You will usually be relieved of your responsibilities when EMS arrives on the scene.

▶ Moving Victims

A victim should not be moved until he or she is ready for transportation to a hospital, if required. A victim should be moved only if there is an immediate danger, such as the following:

- Fire or danger of fire
- Explosives or other hazardous materials
- Impossible to protect the scene from hazards
- Impossible to gain access to other victims in the situation who need lifesaving care (such as in a motor vehicle crash)

Emergency Moves

The major danger in moving a victim quickly is the possibility of aggravating an injury. For a victim lying on the ground, pull the victim in the direction of the long axis of the body to provide as much protection to the spinal cord as possible. Several methods exist for moving victims:

Drags:
- *Shoulder drag:* Use for short distances over a rough surface; stabilize victim's head with your forearms **Figure 14-2** .
- *Ankle drag:* This is the fastest method for a short distance on a smooth surface **Figure 14-3** .
- *Blanket pull:* Roll the victim onto a blanket and pull from behind the victim's head **Figure 14-4** .

One-person moves:
- *Human crutch (one person helps victim walk):* If one leg is injured, help the victim walk on the good leg while you support the injured side **Figure 14-5** .

- *Cradle carry:* Use this method for children and lightweight adults who cannot walk **Figure 14-6** .
- *Fire fighter's carry:* If the victim's injuries permit, you can travel longer distances if you carry the victim over your shoulder **Figure 14-7** .
- *Pack-strap carry:* When injuries make the fire fighter's carry unsafe, this method is better for longer distances **Figure 14-8** .
- *Piggyback carry:* Use this method when the victim cannot walk but can use his or her arms to hang onto the rescuer **Figure 14-9** .

Two-person or three-person moves:
- *Two-person assist:* This method is similar to the human crutch **Figure 14-10** .
- *Two-handed seat carry:* Two people carry the victim **Figure 14-11** .
- *Four-handed seat carry:* This is the easiest two-person carry when no equipment is available and the victim cannot walk but can use his or her arms to hang onto the two rescuers **Figure 14-12** .
- *Extremity carry:* One person supports the victim underneath the victim's arms while the other person supports the victim's legs **Figure 14-13** .
- *Chair carry:* This method is useful for a narrow passage or up or down stairs. Use a sturdy chair that can take the victim's weight **Figure 14-14** .
- *Hammock carry:* Three to six people stand on alternate sides of the injured person and link hands beneath the victim **Figure 14-15** .

Nonemergency Moves

All injured parts should be stabilized before and during moving. If rapid transportation is not needed, it is helpful to practice on another person about the same size as the injured victim.

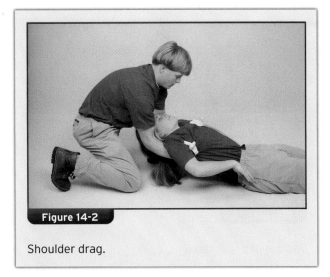

Figure 14-2

Shoulder drag.

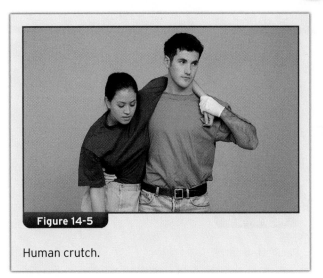

Figure 14-5

Human crutch.

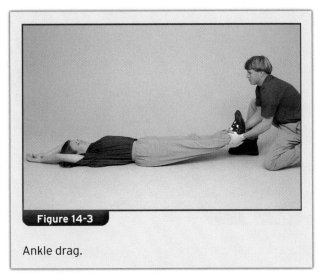

Figure 14-3

Ankle drag.

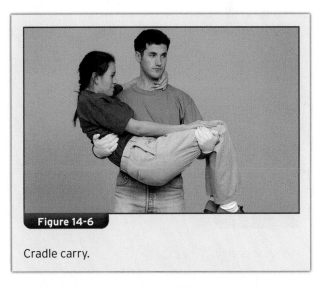

Figure 14-6

Cradle carry.

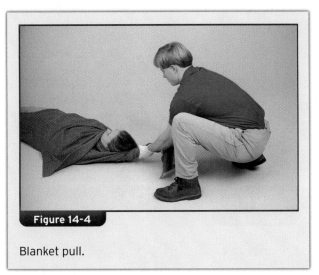

Figure 14-4

Blanket pull.

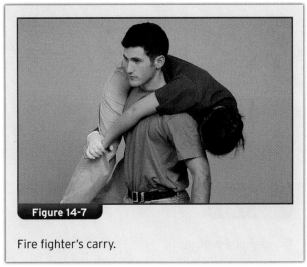

Figure 14-7

Fire fighter's carry.

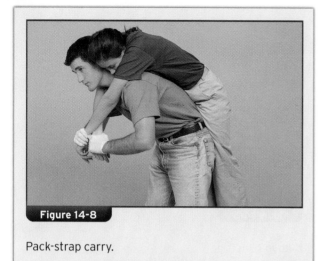

Figure 14-8

Pack-strap carry.

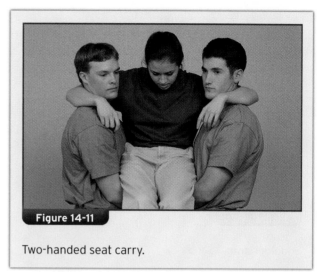

Figure 14-11

Two-handed seat carry.

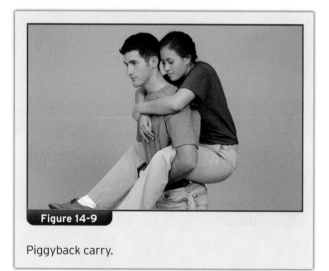

Figure 14-9

Piggyback carry.

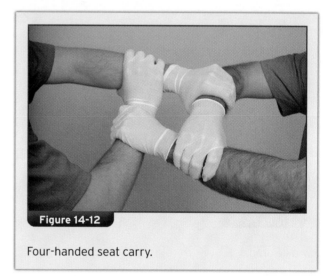

Figure 14-12

Four-handed seat carry.

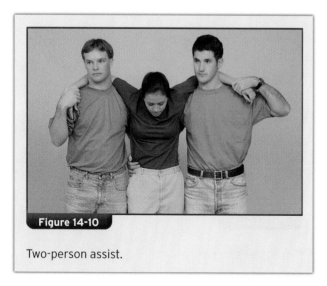

Figure 14-10

Two-person assist.

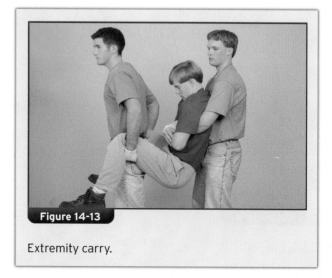

Figure 14-13

Extremity carry.

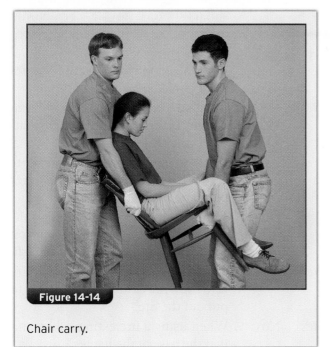

Figure 14-14

Chair carry.

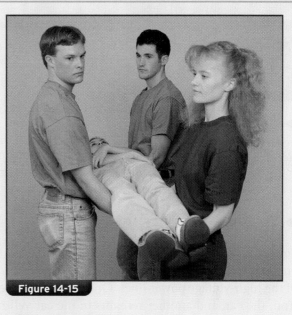

Figure 14-15

Hammock carry.

prep kit

▶ Key Terms

triage The sorting of patients into groups according to the severity of injuries. Used to determine priorities for treatment and transport.

▶ Assessment in Action

You see a single car leave the highway and crash into an electrical power line pole, knocking down some of the high-voltage power lines. One victim is ejected from the car, and another remains in the car yelling for help.

Directions: Circle Yes if you agree with the statement, and circle No if you disagree.

Yes No 1. You should go first to the victim in the car because he or she is pleading for help.

Yes No 2. If one of the victims is in contact with the high-voltage power line, a dry tree branch could be used to move the electrical line.

Yes No 3. Most state laws require a driver of another car witnessing a car crash to stop and render care.

Yes No 4. For the quiet, motionless victim ejected from the car, you should stabilize the head and neck against movement.

Yes No 5. You could consider moving either of the victims if their lives are threatened by a fire.

Answers: 1. No; 2. No; 3. No; 4. Yes; 5. Yes

▶ Check Your Knowledge

Directions: Circle Yes if you agree with the statement, and circle No if you disagree.

Yes No 1. You should attempt to move downed power lines away from a victim by using a broom or other wooden object.

Yes No 2. Strong, unusual odors or clouds of vapor are possible indications of the presence of hazardous materials.

Yes No 3. To keep from becoming trapped while attempting to extinguish a fire, you should always keep a door behind you for rapid exit.

Yes No 4. In a situation involving several victims, those with breathing difficulties need immediate attention.

Yes No 5. A major concern in moving a victim quickly is the possibility of aggravating a spine injury.

Yes No 6. "Row-throw-reach-go" represents the safe order for executing a water rescue.

Yes No 7. In most states, you are legally obligated to stop and give help when you are involved in a motor vehicle crash.

Yes No 8. The first thing to do in case of a fire is to use a fire extinguisher and try to put out the fire.

Yes No 9. When using a fire extinguisher, aim it at the base of the flames.

Yes No 10. When several people are injured, those crying or screaming should receive your attention first.

Answers: 1. No; 2. Yes; 3.Yes; 4. Yes; 5. Yes; 6. No; 7. Yes; 8. No; 9. Yes; 10. No

Meeting OSHA Guidelines

This chapter covers the following *OSHA Best Practices Guide: Fundamentals of a Workplace First Aid Program (2006)*:

3. Assessing the Scene and the Victim(s)
   • Assessing the toxic potential of the environment and the need for respiratory protection;
   • Establishing the presence of a confined space and the need for respiratory protection and specialized training to perform a rescue;
   • Prioritizing care when there are several injured;
   • Indications for and methods of safety moving and rescuing victim(s);
   • Repositioning ill/injured victims to prevent further injury.
4. Responding to Life-Threatening Emergencies
   • Inhaled poisons: carbon monoxide; hydrogen sulfide; smoke; and other chemical fumes, vapors, and gases.
   • Recognizing asphyxiation and the danger of entering a confined space without appropriate respiratory protection.

index

image credits

Chapter 1
Opener Courtesy of Larry Newell; 1-1 Reproduced from U.S. Department of Labor, Bureau of Labor Statistics: Sprains and strains most common workplace injury. Monthly Labor Review, April 1, 2005. Available at: http://www.bls.gov/opub/ted/2005/mar/wk4/art05.htm; 1-2 Vyrostek S.B., Annest J.L., Ryan G.W. Surveillance for Fatal and Nonfatal Injuries - United States, 2001. *MMWR* 53(SSO7); 1-75 (September 3, 2004).; 1-4 Courtesy of Ellis and Associates.

Chapter 2
Opener © Peter Steiner/Alamy Images.

Chapter 3
Opener © Ingram Publishing/age fotostock; 3-2 © Jonathan Noden-Wilkinson/ShutterStock, Inc.; 3-5 Courtesy of MedicAlert Foundation®. © 2006, All Rights Reserved. MedicAlert® is a federally registered trademark and service mark.

Chapter 4
Opener Photographed by Christine McKeen.

Chapter 5
Opener Photographed by Christine McKeen; 5-3 Courtesy of Dey, L.P.

Chapter 7
Opener © Joe Gough/ShutterStock, Inc.

Chapter 8
Opener © Gordon Swanson/ShutterStock, Inc.

Chapter 9
Opener © Christoph & Friends/Das Fotoarchiv/Alamy Images.

Chapter 11
Opener © Stockbyte/Creatas; 11-3 a: © Thomas Photography LLC/Alamy Images; b: © Thomas J. Peterson/ Alamy Images, c: Courtesy of U.S. Fish & Wildlife Service.

Chapter 12
Opener © Jonathan Plant/Alamy Images; 12-2 © AbleStock; 12-5 © Arlindo Ferreira da Silva/ ShutterStock, Inc.; 12-6 © photobar/ShutterStock, Inc.; 12-7 Courtesy of Kenneth Cramer, Monmouth College; 12-9 © Kirubeshwaran/ShutterStock, Inc.; 12-10 a and b: Courtesy of Scott Bauer/USDA.

Chapter 13
Opener © Laura Rauch/AP Photos.

Unless otherwise indicated, photographs are under copyright of Jones and Bartlett Publishers, courtesy of MIEMSS, or the American Academy of Orthopaedic Surgeons.